Look Like Yourself
& Love It!

TRIAD PRESS
Dept. L, P.O. Box 42006, Houston, TX., 77042

Jane Segerstrom's

Look Like Yourself & Love It!

The 4-T Guide to Personal Style

Book Design	Jane Segerstrom
Cover Design & Titles	Keith McNay
Cover Photographer	Chas McGrath
Color Chart Preparation	Betty Towell
Color Separations	San Jacinto Engraving
Monochrome Photographer	Cliff Segerstrom
Illustrator	Gabrielle Manela
Editor	Ruth Nichols
Printer	D. Armstrong Company, Inc.
Binder	Rasch Graphics
Paper	Carnival #60 Vellum
Type	Baskerville 11/13

 TRIAD PRESS, a division of Triad Interests, Inc., Dept. L, Box 42006, Houston, Texas 77042

Library of Congress Cataloging in Publication Data

Segerstrom, Jane.
  Look Like Yourself and Love It!

  Includes index.
  1. Beauty, Personal. 2. Grooming for men. 3. Temperament. 4. Clothing and dress. 5. Men's clothing. I. Nichols, Ruth, 1924- II. Title.
RA776.5.S36   646.7   80-50836
ISBN 0-936740-06-X

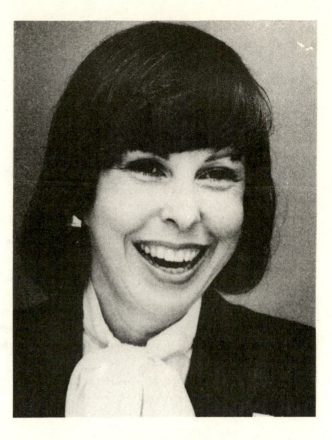

JANE SEGERSTROM, author of *Look Like Yourself & Love It!* is an image specialist, fashion stylist, professional lecturer and television and radio personality.

Influenced by the work of Northern California color analysts Suzanne Caygill, Joan Songer and Don Cardwell, Jane updated her personal style. Then, in T-1 fashion, she proceeded to improve everyone in sight.

Her research has been shared through countless workshops, lectures and guest appearances on radio and television. . . including fifty-five half-hour programs for KGO-TV, San Francisco, which she produced and in which she starred.

Both manufacturers and merchandisers have benefited from her counsel.

Beginning with experience in classroom teaching and adult education, Jane Segerstrom believes in lifelong learning and brings a unique fashion approach to consumers and industry. She currently serves on the National Executive Board of Home Economists in Business.

Native Californians, Cliff and Jane Segerstrom have been married twenty-nine years, have two grown children and reside in Houston.

Contents

Acknowledgments

Much gratitude and personal thanks are due those who contributed time, talent, ideas and support to *Look Like Yourself & Love It!* and to me. They include Doug Brown, Mary Kate Burgess, Mary Ann Caudle, Dick Heckert, Gerald W. Frels, D.D.S., C. Anthony Frilouz, Veranne Graham, Judith H. McQuown, Robert J. Moore, Lillian Riggleman, Brian Rollins, Mary Sears, Olga Sulger, Micki Tichacek, Betty Towell, Connie Malone, Rita Wall, Robert H. Wood, Jr., M.D., the invaluable members of Houston Professional Writers, Dr. Ruth Nichols for kind, helpful editing, and lastly, for years of love and support, my husband, Clifford C. Segerstrom.

Who Are You?

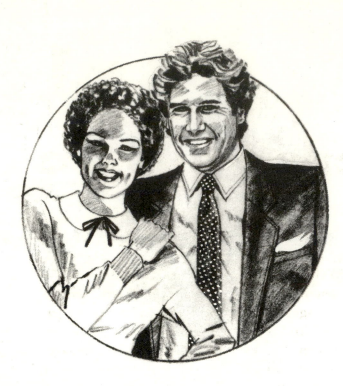

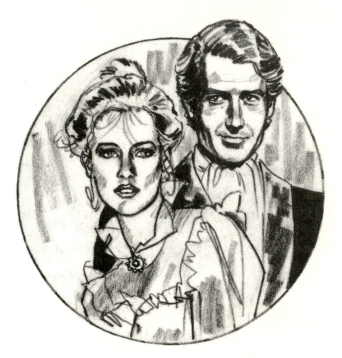

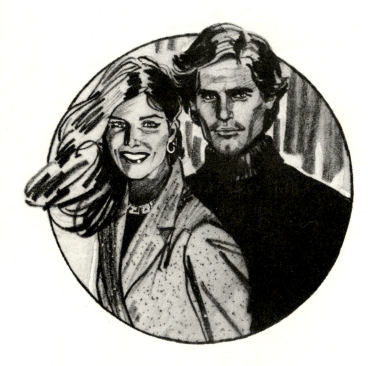

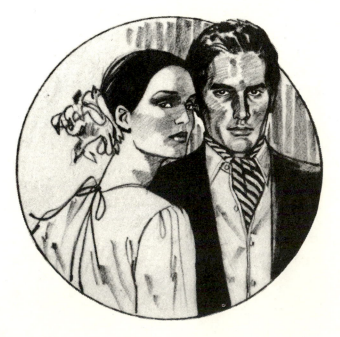

1

From Where You Are

How would *you* describe personal beauty? Until a few years ago I would have described it as a leggy, blue-eyed blonde with thick, curly hair. Interesting, for I described myself as a balloon with short legs, unnoticed eyes and limp, no-color hair. Unaware of my physical assets, I focused on other things, dressing quietly (read that frumpily) and ignoring my exterior. Not until my forties did I realize I had shorted myself, or been shorted, for I AM PRETTY! Why hadn't someone told me? If they had, why hadn't I heard?

Sometime between birth and adulthood, each individual suspects, or knows, his/her appearance is lacking. What the standard or who the judge no one really says. You believe the lie, swallow the poison, and thereafter judge yourself with negatively prejudiced eyes. And extensive evidence supports your false view.

Media proclaims that blonds have more fun; this year's skin is exotic; teeth must be ultra-white for you to be kissable. Families comment on weight, impossible hair, the size of your feet.

You aren't even free to ignore your appearance—the price is too steep. Studies have proven that on blind dates the single criterion for rating men or women is appearance. Personality, intelligence and social skills only begin to count on later meetings.

Other studies indicate attractive people are seen as stronger, kinder and more interesting. They appear to be sexier with more out-going personalities. A child in nursery school will attribute good traits to a nice-looking newcomer and bad traits to a less-attractive stranger. Teachers tend to grade sharp-looking students higher and less-well-groomed ones lower than their accomplishment deserves. Lighter sentences and more ready parole are given to handsome, well-groomed felons . . . stiffer sentences to those less visually pleasing.

How do you get *from where you are* to looking handsome or pretty? Begin by walking down a busy street and collecting impressions of those you pass. You may find only one person out of fifty projecting more than a blur. That one individual may be obviously handicapped, outlandishly dressed or unusually handsome. Rare the man or woman who turns heads because he or she looks superb.

One who *blurs* broadcasts too-many differing impressions. Each individual choice of garment, style, color, texture, hair, makeup, accessory makes a statement. Unfortunately, the statements are contradictory—eradicating, not illuminating. Should you wish to know the individual, you feel like asking the real Sue or Jim to please identify herself/himself.

I've a warm kinship with *one who blurs*, for until recently that description fit me. The mixed-image person may be ultra busy, service oriented, physically or mentally ill, lacking funds, needing inspiration or missing vital information. Whatever, if you're *one who blurs*, you're robbing yourself.

The secret to projecting a striking look doesn't require regular features or a perfect physique, fortunately. Your face and body plus interest in improving yourself and knowledge of how to proceed is all you need. This book shares information never previously available. The interest you must supply yourself; but you'll have plenty if you're as tired as I was of looking and feeling plain.

Hundreds of men and women have switched from ordinary to great and loved their transformation. They used my techniques. You can, too.

Have I mentioned that wriggling out of your old image requires work? I should, for valuable possessions, like your new look, must be paid for. Your new image requires, for openers, giving up downgrading yourself. It may be difficult. You've devoted years to the put-self-down game. But you'll find the results invaluable, considering your bonus is a lifetime's enjoyment of your "special" look. Get a roommate, spouse, or friend to signal whenever you utter a "dumb me" expression. Give your new image a chance.

Looking stunning requires discipline. You'll soon select only those garments and accessories which are personally becoming and reject those merely beautiful, kicky or "in." Your new clothes will highlight your bone structure, personality and coloring—not denying what you are but displaying it. When fashion authorities decide this or that is perfect for brownettes, you won't believe it. Brownettes differ too much for generalizations.

Each person faces a thousand new ideas each season: ways to wear a handkerchief or tie a scarf, kinds and widths of belts, colors, textures and prints, and various shapes including hairstyles. One idea out of the whole catalog may be perfect for you, another for me. To select that perfect one and ignore the others must become your goal.

Simple rules and guidelines are what I needed and found. Here are stories of four people who also found those rules and guidelines and learned to capitalize on their looks.

— JOY —

Middle-aged Joy was average height, but, like many, carried twenty extra pounds on her small-boned frame. A home economist, she sewed beautifully, but her clothing looked dowdy. She'd tried vivid, pale and grayed colorations. None became her, so she wore neutrals. Joy had surrendered her childish enthusiasm after judging it inappropriate to both her age and her roles of wife, mother and teacher. Over the years she learned to accept her interior, but her exterior received little time or attention. She had retired from the appearance game—no contest.

Through this theory Joy discovered her best look is young, pretty and doll-like. With her excess weight gone (valuing herself made those pounds go more easily) small bones became an asset. She learned to wear crisp, smooth fabrics; clear, bright colors; and small scale, round-shaped detailing on necklines, collars, lapels, buttons, buckles, and jewelry. Her baby-fine hair is blunt cut and blown dry in a style that emphasizes her eyes.

Joy is happily gathering compliments, such as, "Those can't be your children. You're not old enough." "You have fantastic eyes, really sparkling!" "I love you in those colors—would never have thought to put them together." And one of the loveliest, "You're so slim and little—surely you never had a weight problem."

Feeling pretty and girlish, Joy considers it wasteful not to have discovered herself earlier. But her long-suppressed animation comes bubbling forth with the words, "I'm delighted to be me, at long last."

— HANK —

Hank was a slim, wiry five-feet-seven. His dark-blonde hair, hazel eyes and heavily-textured skin failed to please him. He needed to be tall and dark to make the impression he wanted. Hank had ambition and drive, and he was on the corporate ladder, but key people failed to notice.

Hank's clothes were expensive and in excellent taste. He typically wore a grey pin-stripe suit with a white shirt and maroon tie, or a navy blazer-suit with a light-blue and white striped shirt and a navy and red polka-dot tie.

Once Hank discovered how to make his coloring and bone structure an asset, he proceeded to choose clothing from a different perspective.

He now wears gauzy or handwoven shirts in earthtones. His tweed, herringbone and plaid suits are subtle, but the lapels are sharp and the pocket detailing—angular. Buttons are no longer classic; now they're rough-textured metal, bone or woven leather. He chooses paisley, zigzags and diagonally-striped patterns for ties.

While Hank's former clothes unflatteringly emphasized his rough skin and angular features, his new clothes minimize facial irregularities and maximize strength.

Hank also uses color to regulate how others see him, a valuable bonus. He can choose to appear either highly masculine, dramatic, comfortable or supportive. His look is now one of virility and strength—image matching man.

The dramatic improvement in Hank's dress boosted his ego, intrigued his business associates and raised his income. Hank even gained a new account without saying a word. The prospect said, "Anyone looking as good as you do must have something going for him."

— PHILIP —

Philip was tall and thin with long, slender hands and feet. His father had wanted Philip to be a man's man: aggressive, strong and sports-loving. He was, instead, sensitive, gentle and introspective. As a child he hid from or suffered the rough games and sports which delighted his peers. As an adult he was artistic and spiritual, not at all his father's man. Measured against our culture's standard of maleness he flunked the test, questioned his own manhood and considered himself a failure.

Now Philip accepts his personal worth. He realizes his tastes and temperament are shared by many well-adjusted men and women, and he feels "okay" being who he is. Fear left when understanding arrived.

Philip looks different, too, for he chooses soft colors such as taupe, dove grey, greyed-green, gentle yellow, mauve or lavender. He wears variations of one color from head to toe, keeping contrast to a minimum. His is a romantic image, reminiscent of a more-cultured era.

His wardrobe contains English-cut suits of soft luxurious fabrics, elegant dress boots, silk ascots and a marvelous plum-velvet smoking jacket. His jewelry choices are highly refined: for instance, pearl studs and cufflinks of brushed-silver ovals. Looking at Philip you envision a cavalier with plumed hat, buckled knee britches and a sword at his side. He's a highly-prized androgenous man.

— NORMA —

Norma, at sixteen, was different. She seemed older, quieter and more of an introvert than her friends. They loved chattering about clothes, boys and sports. She loved books. Her parents, strong extroverts, wanted a happy, popular daughter. They bought pretty, girlish clothes which Norma's friends adored. Norma thought the clothes pretty, too; but when she tried them on, she looked even more different. They seemed to belong to someone else. She dressed as other girls dressed, yet it wasn't becoming. Why?

Norma's best look is a beautiful one, totally understated; no frills, trims or applied design. Since her dark hair and eyes contrast with the white oval of her face, she wears clothing with the simplest of lines. But nothing drab for her. Her colors are brilliant or sharply black or white. Her facial contrast is exciting enough to supply all the POW one could wish. Her vivid colors highlight—never upstage.

Norma's selections are the same general type as those of her friends, but now Norma's clothes belong to her. Her jeans aren't blue denim; they're velveteen or the finest-wale corduroy. Her tops are simple: tee shirts with oval necklines, turtlenecks or classic shirts—all in fine fabrics. She wears ascots, not bows, and straight skirts, not dirndls. She chooses smooth fabrics, not textures, prints or tweeds. She still looks unlike her contemporaries, but she looks cool and beautiful.

Norma realizes that in a few years her beauty will mature and she will be outstanding. What a wonderful way to look and feel at sixteen!

Would you like to discover yourself, your own best look? Would you like to know what to choose and what not to choose when you're facing a myriad of choices? Would you like to express a perfect image, to LOOK LIKE YOURSELF AND LOVE IT? Then check the appropriate places.

yes	no	
_____	_____	I have the desire.
_____	_____	I'm willing to try something new.
_____	_____	I'll consider the ideas in this book.

If "Yes" is your answer, then come on . . .

2

Your Personality

Granted, you are unique. Millions of categories would be insufficient to catalog everyone, yet fewer than a million must be used if you're to understand your best image and learn how to achieve it.

This system places each individual in one of four major groups. But the Four Types of categories used within this book have a 2,000-year precedent.

— HIPPOCRATES TO LAHAYE —

Hippocrates, the father of modern medicine, lived 400 years before Christ. In an age of superstition he believed in facts. He taught that people could be classified into four distinct groups according to their personalities or temperaments. Those groupings were called: Sanguine, Melancholy, Choleric and Phlegmatic. Hippocrates named the groups after the four "humors" of the body: blood, black bile, yellow bile and phlegm, which he believed to be responsible for the variations in temperament. Scientists have long since discarded the possibility that body fluids are responsible for personality variations, but the field of biochemistry is so new the real causes are yet to be isolated.

A San Diego minister/author, Tim LaHaye, uses Hippocrates' categories in counseling. By helping his counselees recognize how they fit into the four categories, LaHaye helps each person grow in self-understanding. His parishioners learn to understand their own strengths and weaknesses and to accept and even anticipate the behavior of those who function differently from themselves. This has proven itself to be a beautiful tool for marriage partners, parents, or any two people brought closely together.

Let's change Hippocrates' ungraceful terms to simpler ones. It's doubtful if anyone would really like to be called Melancholic or Choleric; so let's use Type One, Type Two, Type Three, and Type Four, or T-1, T-2, T-3, and T-4.

Locate yourself in the following descriptions.

With which group do you most identify?

— TYPE ONE PERSONALITY —

Vivacious describes them. They're cheerleader types, hungry for life. Active sports, projects and causes alternate with people and parties to totally engage them. Type Ones' openness attracts both sexes, and facility with words assures an audience. Their animated description of "schussing down the slope" or "landing the *big* one" charms admirers and earns the reputation of entertaining storytellers.

Type Ones sometimes come on too strong, dominate the conversation and exaggerate the truth; but their warmth and sympathy counterbalance. They speak without thinking—verbally destructive as a frisky puppy in an antique-filled room—but their charm, like the puppy's, earns quick forgiveness.

Often restless, undisciplined and easily distracted, Type Ones may be careless with possessions and unaware of discarded clothing draping furniture and floors.

Last week's thrilling new project is rarely today's excitement, for enthusiasm is T-1's long suit while persistence is their void. They're experimental and stimulating lovers, but not always faithful.

Emotions sweep T-1s from bubbling high spirits to wracking sobs. They may seem phony with their swift shifts, but they genuinely FEEL. Empathetic and easily moved, T-1s love you more and forget you faster than any other type.

But, don't be mislead. Not all T-1s are mercurial. Within this category live straightforward citizens who are obviously alert but quieter, the no frills, no nonsense type. Also included are the innocents and ingenues aged four to ninety-four.

Type Ones test high in persuasion, the trait most needed in sales, service, and teaching.

A typical T-1 skips through life slightly airborne, one hand clasping a red balloon, the other a newly-made friend. He displays a big grin and is, of course, talking.

# # # # #

Do YOU have a Type One personality? Underline the words on the following checklist that pertain to you. Don't worry if you don't relate to any of the words, there are three more lists. Consider, also, having a close friend check the lists for you. Friends often supply a version of you more enlightening and accurate than your own. Grab a pencil and *underline*.

T-1 CHECKLIST A

adaptable	eager	helpful	outspoken
animated	earnest	imaginative	playful
bright	eloquent	impulsive	refreshing
candid	emotional	inconsistent	restless
carefree	enthusiastic	innocent	simple
casual	flirtatious	lively	sincere
changeable	forgetful	loveable	sociable
cheerful	free	mischievous	sunny
child-like	fresh	naive	talkative
charming	friendly	open	tender
clean-cut	generous	opportunistic	uninhibited
compassionate	genuine	optimistic	warm
curious	grinning	outdoorsy	wholesome
direct	gullible	out-going	youthful

Count the number of underlined words.
Write your total for T-1 CHECKLIST A here

22 .

— TYPE TWO PERSONALITY —

Type Twos are sensitive and gifted. Their analytical ability and introspection find creative expression in fields such as invention, science, religion, philosophy, literature, arts, photography, music, drama and design—including make-up, hair, costume, sets and interiors. They're quiet, complex, gentle . . . true gentlemen or lovely ladies with all the positive meanings those terms have ever possessed. One would think these gifted people stepped out of a slower-paced, more elegant and graceful era. Their ideal picnic would include crystal stemware for the wine and a long floaty dress for the lady.

T-2s love comfort and beauty. They collect the exquisite for home or apartment and, if possible, drive a handsome, well-appointed, air-conditioned car. These inactive souls prefer being comfortably seated or reclined to standing or moving.

Type Twos will analyze a person with so penetrating a gaze he'll feel naked and unable to dissemble. Fortunately, appreciation for beauty and truth plus love and acceptance join in that analysis; so the object of their gaze is, in the next instant, freed and relaxed, knowing his uniqueness is understood and valued.

These gentle T-2s are loyal friends, a precious gift. They are gracious hosts, extending all courtesies, but their tendency toward moodiness, self-pity, and depression can block their hospitality. These perfectionists are private, suffering people. More geniuses and more suicides come from this group than from any other. Up, they radiate brilliance; down, they're critical, self-centered, and pessimistic. Rarely are T-2s with the norm.

Occasionally this group's super-sensitive antennae pick up negative vibrations from brusque salespersons or thoughtless acquaintances and feelings are bruised. Since obvious outlets for anger are rarely used, hurts may smolder for years. Having a score of ninety-eight successes to two failures, T-2s tend to focus on the failures, a debilitating habit and one that needs fighting.

Although T-2s may appear weak, they actually are strong. Their struggle to focus creatively outward instead of destructively inward often leads to a deep personal faith, one which undergirds and redirects energies.

# # # # #

Are you a Type Two? Underline those words which apply to you. Don't be concerned with how few or how many words you underline in this, or any other list. Don't be modest either; modesty can keep you from discovering *you*.

T-2 CHECKLIST A

abstract	expensive	long-suffering	refined
aristocratic	faithful	loving	reflective
artistic	fearful	loyal	reserved
comforting	genial	meditating	romantic
conscientious	gentle	melancholy	sensitive
creative	gifted	mysterious	sentimental
cultured	graceful	paranoid	smooth
dedicated	honest	perfectionistic	soft-spoken
devoted	idealistic	pessimistic	sophisticated
dignified	imaginative	philosophical	spiritual
discerning	impractical	pliable	supportive
elegant	intense	precise	talented
elusive	inventive	profound	tender
emotional	learned	quiet	truthful

Count the number of words you've underlined. Write your total for **T-2 CHECKLIST A** here ___24___.

Just as Types One and Two share a gentle receptiveness, Types Three and Four share objectivity and a bent for problem solving. It's as though T-1s and T-2s, whatever their gender, have qualities traditionally considered more feminine, while T-3s and T-4s have qualities generally considered more masculine.

— TYPE THREE PERSONALITY —

Type Threes are direct and goal oriented. They confidently determine their target and aggressively reach it. With unlimited energy as propulsion, T-3s' progress is inevitable as dawn—non-blocked by people, ideas or circumstances. Being practical and single of purpose, their goal is the top. Boardrooms bulge with Type Threes.

Highly organized, yet often lacking analytical reasoning, T-3s approach everything from a utilitarian viewpoint, asking, "How does or will this affect me?" They rarely waste time on doubt or reflection and confidently know *their* way is best.

The male T-3, like the movie hero, is a bold leader, fearless and fast-on-the-draw. He's chasing the villain, solving the problem and overcoming the obstacle. Women fall at his feet or into his bed. Remind you of James Bond?

Once, all young males were trained to act "like BIG boys" . . . sticking-up for their rights . . . not crying when hurt. Some found it difficult, but not the fortunate young Type Three. His traits had been used as the standard.

T-3 females share the strengths of T-3 males but, unfortunately, not their supportive patterning. Traditionally, females have been taught to be accepters, not defenders of their rights nor ambitious for the top. It has hurt no one worse than the Southern, female T-3.

A Type Three from Alabama was carefully reared to be a "lady." She calls it playing *Magnolia Blossom*. First her father and then her husband enjoyed/demanded such a role to emphasize their maleness. She feels that denying her personality was too costly . . . sees a psychiatrist regularly. She's not a *Magnolia Blossom* but a *Tigress*.

Difficulties occur when non-Southern T-3 females marry T-2 males. Growth and understanding are necessary to escape the domineering wife/Milquetoast husband caricature.

Character flaws common to Type Threes include boredom with details, pride, harshness and obsession with a single viewpoint. Impervious to others' feelings, they leave bodies behind as they stride ahead. Violent anger may accompany T-3's being blocked and they may seem domineering, sarcastic, and feel unneedful of God or man.

T-3s of both sexes are naturally sensuous and earthy. The unbuttoned shirt is as natural to them as the buttoned-up is to others. An air of danger surrounds them . . . their sexual energy only partially hidden.

\# \# \# \# \#

Are you a Type Three? To find out, underline those words which apply to you.

T-3 CHECKLIST A

✓able	✓determined	?goal-oriented	✓productive
absorbed	direct	✓guarded	✓proud
aggressive	dominating	hard-headed	✓resistant
✓alert	dramatic	impetuous	✓self-sufficient
authoritative	driving	insensitive	sensuous
bold	dynamic	intense	sharp
✓businesslike	earthy ?	intriguing	spirited
colorful	✓energetic	✓mature	stern
competitive	exciting ?	mysterious	stubborn
confident ?	exotic	opportunistic	sturdy
✓controlled	explosive	✓optimistic	successful
daring	fiery	✓outdoorsy	tough-skinned
decisive	✓firm	powerful	unafraid
demanding	forceful	✓practical	vivid

Count the number of underlined words.
Write your total for T-3 CHECKLIST A here

_16_.

— TYPE FOUR PERSONALITY —

Type Fours are clear-headed and non-emotional. They survey the entire scene before making decisions. Dependably and methodically performing each task, T-4s work quietly and efficiently. They're cool, practical and precise—totally unflappable.

Type Fours are neat about their person and possessions; and, like T-2s, T-4s aim for perfection. They, too, love beautiful possessions, luxurious clothes and perfectly prepared food. They're good friends but perhaps not so ready to lay-down-their life as is T-2.

Because of clear objectivity, T-4s make excellent counselors. They listen quietly before pinpointing difficulties. They're diplomatic, easy-going, and have a delightful sense of humor. Theirs is a fine stabilizing presence. No impetuous words flow from these super-introverts. They're amazingly close-mouthed about themselves and their affairs.

Weaknesses common to Type Fours are slowness and laziness. They often retreat from activity, refusing involvement and resisting change. Selfishness and stubbornness need to be guarded against. While remaining stoically unflappable they can use wit and insight to tease an acquaintance into defenselessness. They're Godlike beings, upon Olympus, viewing human foibles from a safe distance.

Type Fours, like Type Threes, exhibit a more masculine or direct manner. While they share this similarity, they are dissimilar in relative temperature. T-4 is cool where T-3 is warm. T-4 seems to be saying, "I want to be alone," while T-3's message is, "Come 'onna my house."

These intellectuals often choose other T-4s as marriage partners. They excel in positions of authority but won't deliberately seek such a position. Even small companies should have at least one T-4 employee to lend stability and balance.

# # # # #

Is it possible that you're a Type Four? Underline the following words that apply to you. Don't be surprised if you have underlined words in each of the four categories. I've never met anyone who underlines words in only one list.

accurate efficient mysterious stubborn
brilliant exact objective sympathetic
calm good natured observant teasing
capable gracious passive thrifty
civilized honorable perfectionist timeless
classic humorous polished tranquil
conservative immaculate practical unbelieving
controlled impartial principled unemotional
cool impressive reasonable unmotivated
critical incisive refined vivid
dignified intelligent responsible well-bred
diplomatic just serene well-liked
direct magnetic self-protective well-read
dramatic methodical slow witty

Count the number of words you've underlined. Write your total for T-4 CHECKLIST
A here ___33___.

A tally sheet is available on page 42. Enter your totals from the four checklists in the appropriate boxes. Relax, there are no wrong combinations. You may have underlined only a few words or a great many. Underlined words may have been overwhelmingly one type, evenly divided between the four, or with varying amounts in each. You can't fail this test. You're unique, after all, and not an android with a programmed personality.

Thankfully, no harmony or type is better or worse than another. Each is different. In the same way, you aren't supremely blessed or severely handicapped solely by the personality you inherited. You may be handicapped with your attitude about yourself, but not with your God-given personality. The potential to be a beautiful person resides within you. To reach that potential you must first accept yourself where you are. The last two sentences are meant to be read twice.

No harmony is free from potential negative traits just as no individual is totally free from his negative side. Understanding your hazards should alert you to danger. Overcoming negatives requires strength, but it develops strength, as well. Every bad habit we successfully break makes it easier to break the next one.

The Temperament Traits chart on the next page can be a second tool for determining your personality. Underline the work you do, or would like to do, and any traits which pertain to you. Notice that favorable traits are outside the circle, less flattering ones inside. Count the number underlined in each numbered section and record here and under Checklist B on page 42.

CHECKLIST B

1. _____5_____ 2. _____4____ 3. _____6_____ 4. _____9_____

One additional way to classify your personality uses the psychological terms introvert and extrovert.

An *introvert* concentrates on his own thoughts and feelings. He turns mental interests away from persons and events of the outer world, preferring the inner world of private thoughts.

An *extrovert* directs interests and energies toward activities, people, and events of the outer world. He may be unaware of his interior world for long periods.

Those who are normal balance between the two parts, but the scales generally are weighted a bit heavier on one side than the other. Too wide a swing away from balance may indicate neurosis.

Can you decide which represents you? Puzzle it out, then record your results here and as directed on the Tally Sheet on page 42.

CHECKLIST C

_____Introvert   _____Extrovert

TEMPERAMENT TRAITS

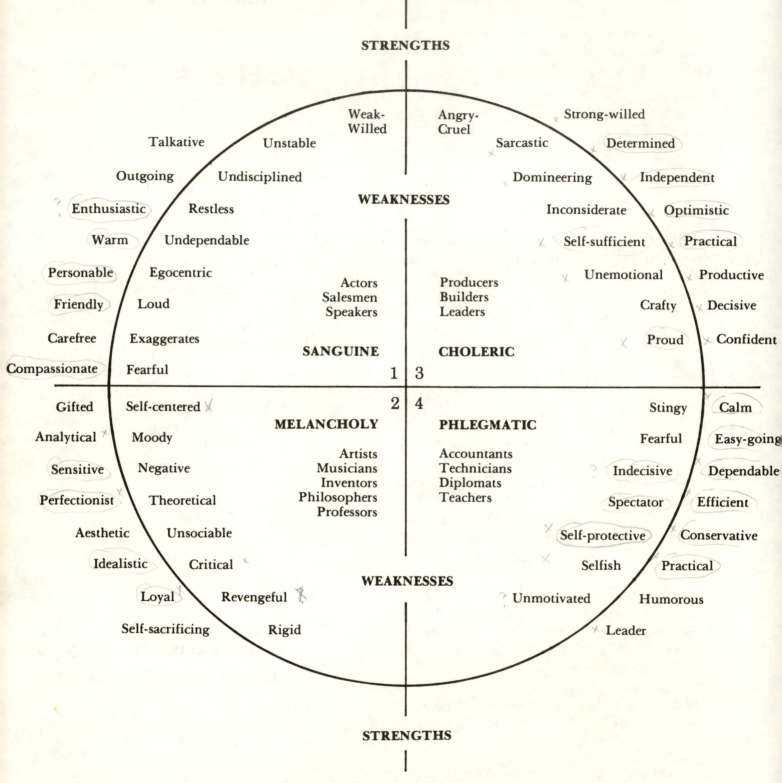

STRENGTHS

WEAKNESSES

Weak-Willed — Angry-Cruel

Talkative — Unstable — Strong-willed

Outgoing — Undisciplined — Sarcastic — Determined

Enthusiastic — Restless — Domineering — Independent

Warm — Undependable — Inconsiderate — Optimistic

Personable — Egocentric — Self-sufficient — Practical

Friendly — Loud — Unemotional — Productive

Carefree — Exaggerates — Crafty — Decisive

Compassionate — Fearful — Proud — Confident

SANGUINE | **CHOLERIC**

Actors — Producers
Salesmen — Builders
Speakers — Leaders

1 | 3
2 | 4

MELANCHOLY | **PHLEGMATIC**

Gifted — Self-centered — Stingy — Calm

Analytical — Moody — Fearful — Easy-going

Sensitive — Negative — Indecisive — Dependable

Perfectionist — Theoretical — Spectator — Efficient

Aesthetic — Unsociable — Self-protective — Conservative

Idealistic — Critical — Selfish — Practical

Loyal — Revengeful — Unmotivated — Humorous

Self-sacrificing — Rigid — Leader

Artists — Accountants
Musicians — Technicians
Inventors — Diplomats
Philosophers — Teachers
Professors

WEAKNESSES

STRENGTHS

Source: *Transformed Temperaments*, Tim
LaHaye, Tyndale House Publishers, 1971.

3

Your Appearance

Personality is a useful tool for indicating one's Type, but appearance is equally effective. If the two were in opposition we'd have a dilemma, but they aren't. Recent independent research by Frances Quinn, Suzanne Caygill, Joan Songer and Don Cardwell in the San Francisco Bay area has proven one's coloring, bone structure and personality mutually reinforcing. You're made right.

Classifying oneself by appearance is possible anytime following the fourth birthday. Each person will remain in one classification throughout life, so the earlier one can "know their type," the better. Thousands of dollars in mistaken and inappropriate purchases can be saved. But more important, self-knowledge frees the spirit.

You might think each race fits neatly into one of the four groups, but they don't. Each race has members in all four divisions. Some orientals look exotic, but others appear fragile, jolly or striking.

Since a number of perceptive individuals can "type" a child or adult, the ability could be a common one. But no. The capacity to "see what you look at" varies widely. Some individuals can't distinguish fine differences and never develop that skill. Others have unsuspected aptitudes which they need to expand. All skills are developed with exercise and this one is no exception.

Play the "What is she?" "What is he?" game when you can observe others, unobserved. The goal is to place each individual in one of the four Types. But a warning—putting someone in the wrong group won't matter when you keep your results to yourself. It's harmful when you're wrong and you tell them. *Keep all guesses private!*

How do you determine in which Type they, or you, belong? These are the characteristics the "Pros" look for . . .

— TYPE ONE APPEARANCE —

Type Ones look smooth and rounded. Appearing younger than their years, T-1s' faces, cheeks, eyes and figures are predominately curved. With short or upturned noses, rosebud lips and curly hair, they move freely, quickly, impulsively. Their speech is soft and rapid.

T-1s' skin may be light as a blue-eyed blonde's or dark as a chocolate, but creamy light seems to shine through it. They look great with tans (the WORST thing you can do to your skin). Type Ones' hair color may range from white to black through all the grays, yellows, reds and browns. Theirs is a fresh, clean quality, the American girl or boy look, the perpetual ingenue. Or think Scandinavian.

One immediate tipoff to this harmony is the grin which lights the face. T-1s seem to be bursting with health and good spirits.

# # # # #

Reread T-1's description and *underline* the words that pertain to you, if any. Count the number of underlined ideas and record your results here and on page 42.

T-1 CHECKLIST D _____.

The following celebrities are examples of T-1s. They vary in coloring, sex, age and race, but all share a young look. *Underline* those stars you resemble or relate to.

T-1 CHECKLIST E

Pearl Bailey	Johnny Carson
Carol Burnett	Shaun Cassidy
Bo Derek	John Davidson
Chris Evert Lloyd	John Denver
Goldie Hawn	Phil Donahue
Liza Minelli	Michael Landon
Marie Osmond	Rich Little
Dolly Parton	Donnie Osmond
Cheryl Tiegs	Ryan O'Neal
Cindy Williams	Flip Wilson

Count the number of names you have underlined. Record that number here and on page 42.

T-1 CHECKLIST E _____.

— TYPE TWO APPEARANCE —

Type Twos have a gentle, ageless appearance. Although rarely pretty as children, they mature into a delicate beauty. Bodies are more elongated than T-1s', foreheads more generous, chins straighter or receding and features more refined. Hands and feet of Type Twos are long and aristocratic with gently tapering fingers and toes—gracefully designed for artistic endeavors and expensive shoes.

Type Two's quiet coloring matches soft voices and non-flashy personalities. Their eyes are a grayed form of many different color possibilities from dark to light. Teeth are creamy, skins are whiter or grayer in varying values to very dark and hair is silky-fine with ash undertones. Males of this group look wonderful with well-trimmed facial hair.

Type Twos at a party will be by themselves or talking with one other person. They shun the limelight and will be the last ones you notice.

# # # # #

Reread this section and *underline* the descriptions that pertain to you, if any. Count the number of underlined ideas and record your results here and on page 42.

T-2 CHECKLIST D _____.

The following celebrities are examples of T-2s. They also vary in coloring, sex, age, and race; but their image is romantic. *Underline* those stars you resemble or relate to.

T-2 CHECKLIST E

Marisa Berenson	Alan Arkin
Queen Elizabeth	Warren Beatty
Joan Fontaine	Prince Charles
Greta Garbo	Clint Eastwood
Princess Grace	Marcel Marceau
Barbara Hershey	Jim McKay
Olivia Hussey	Sylvester Stallone
Lauren Hutton	John Travolta
Dina Merrill	Michael York
Joanne Woodward	Robin Williams

Count the number of names you've underlined. Record that number here and on page 42.

T-2 CHECKLIST E _____.

— TYPE THREE APPEARANCE —

Type Threes are more earthy, exotic or dangerous than the other types. Features have more angularity and sharpness, and coloring is warmer with undertones of black, brown or yellow. They have coarser hair than T-2s' and rough textured skin. When hair grays it becomes multi-colored like a rich, wonderful tweed. Eyes may be set obliquely or deeply and their color is blue-green to black, most often brown, but *never clear blue.* Lashes sometimes grow straight down. Brows may be bushy or angular. Large, aquiline, convex-curved or flared-nostriled noses may grace these interesting faces. Cheekbones are often high above flat cheeks. Jaws may be sharp or jutting. Bones are often large, shoulders broad.

T-3 voices are positive, strong, deep and, occasionally, loud. Stride is either long and confident or sensuous. You can't miss seeing these rough, warm, sexy powerhouses.

# # # # #

Reread this section and *underline* the descriptions that pertain to you, if any. Count the number of underlined ideas and record your results here and on page 42.

T-3 CHECKLIST D _____.

The following celebrities are examples of T-3s. They vary in coloring, sex, age and race, but all share a look of strength. *Underline* those you resemble or relate to.

T-3 CHECKLIST E

Rosie Casals	Charles Bronson
Lena Horne	Sammy Davis, Jr.
Glenda Jackson	Peter Falk
Cloris Leachman	Walter Matthau
Sophia Loren	Lee Marvin
Penny Marshall	Joe Namath
Charlotte Rampling	Jack Nicholson
Barbra Streisand	Anthony Quinn
Barbara Walters	Burt Reynolds
Raquel Welch	John Wayne

Count the number of names you've underlined. Record that number here and on page 42.

T-3 CHECKLIST E _____.

— TYPE FOUR APPEARANCE —

Type Fours are beautiful. Their perfection of feature plus, contrasting darkness/light-ness immediately draws attention. Eyes of this group are deep shades of blue, green, brown, or gray. Both whites of eyes and teeth are whiter than those of the other groups. T-4s' smooth skin is white as porcelain, jet black, creamy yellow or clear brown. Hair is dark; but when it turns, it's snowy white. Faces are elongated ovals with well-proportioned features which contribute to a flowing, finely-sculptured look. Hands and feet are slim and graceful.

Type Fours give the appearance of wealth and their cool, detached, formal-yet-gracious manner matches. They speak clearly, walk erectly and gracefully, and are more nearly perfect in visual design than any other group.

# # # # #

Reread this section and underline the descriptions that pertain to you, if any. Count the number of underlined ideas and record your results here and on page 42.

T-4 CHECKLIST D _____.

The following celebrities are examples of T-4s. They vary in coloring, sex, age and race, but all share an inner coolness. *Underline* those you resemble or relate to.

T-4 CHECKLIST E

Diahann Carroll	Tony Curtis
Cher	Robert DeNiro
Peggy Fleming	Erik Estrada
Crystal Gayle	James Garner
Audrey Hepburn	George Hamilton
Mary McFadden	Rock Hudson
France Nuyen	Anthony Newley
Jackie Onassis	Anthony Perkins
Jaclyn Smith	Sidney Poitier
Liz Taylor	Omar Sharif

Count the number of names you've underlined. Record that number here and on page 42.

T-4 CHECKLIST E _____.

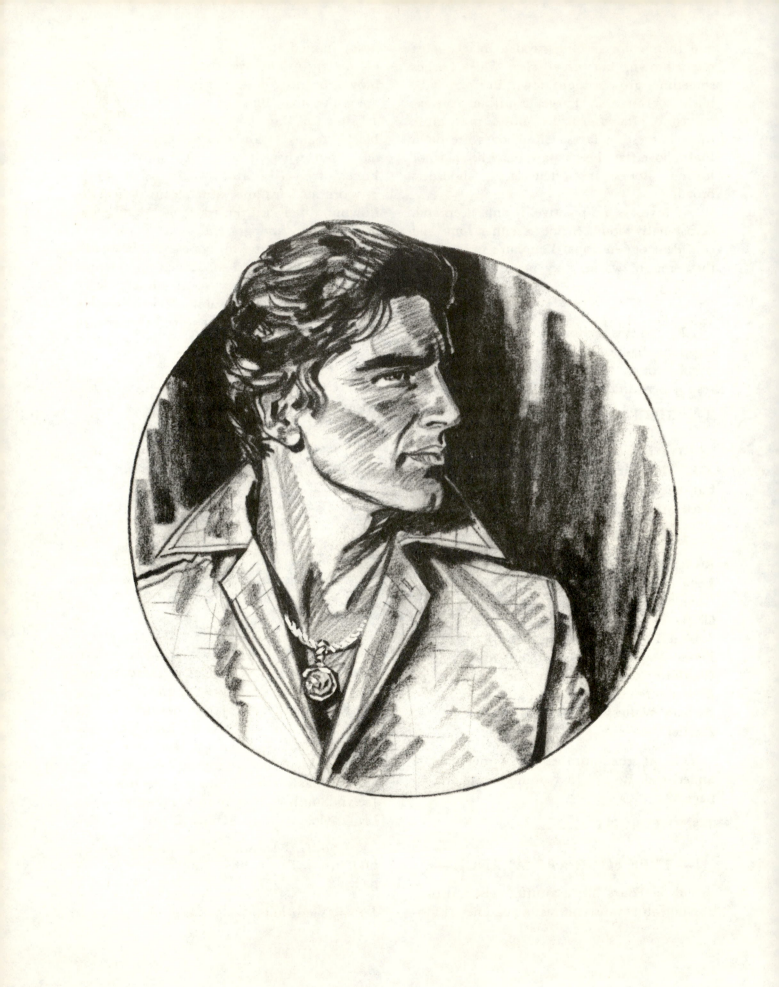

4

Your Coloring

Do you conveniently fit one of the four categories? Lucky you! If you don't, relax. You're not alone. Most people are so complex their physical characteristics and personalities fall under more than one type—occasionally under three or four. You won't be left drawing straws, fortunately. There is one last determiner.

A test to break your deadlock—the most valuable test you can take—determines your exact coloring plus the colors that make you look "great." This test should remove doubts and tip the scales to one specific Type or the other. The tool you develop will be helpful all your life in selecting clothing, accessories, home decor, boat and car colors.

This clothing tool, or color stick, is your own coloring reduced to a cardboard "key" that you use objectively to select "super" colors, personally exciting ones. By limiting your color choices to those working *for* you, you'll find fantastic selections for yourself and, rather neatly, place yourself in one of the four categories.

Personal coloring is composed of four parts: hair, eyes, skin and liptone. All four must be considered when determining a color's becomingness. All four must be your *natural* coloring, as well. Changes in hair via bleach, dye, tint, or frost obscure your look, as do *tinted* contact lenses, as does a *corrective* makeup color, as does a *wrong* lipstick. You match yourself, not a painted doll ... if you would look wonderful.

People are often blind to *specific* shades, for they don't look specifically. They see in generalizations, a car, instead of the specific, a white Volkswagen "bug" with ski rack. You need to see specific colors. Look intently at each of the colors which make up *your* facial coloring: hair, eyes, skin and liptone. When you see each color clearly you can begin to relate your hair color in the mirror to a similar shade on a magazine page, a paint store color chip or a fabric swatch. When you have located and isolated those four colors which represent your face, you'll have an increased objectivity and appreciation of self. They're *always* a beautiful collage. You'll also have supplied yourself with an invaluable tool for choosing clothing.

A specific color is identified by its three distinct characteristics: hue, value and intensity. To match a color you need to be certain it is similar in all three aspects. *Hue* is the color designation, such as reddish-brown or greenish-brown. *Value* is the darkness or lightness, such as chocolate brown or pale beige. *Intensity* is the brightness or dullness, such as vivid rust or muted red-brown.

Now actively seek color samples similar to your hair, eyes, skin and lips. If you can't find an exact match, choose samples that come as close as possible. You can "bracket" a color by using two colors that are very near, one on each side. Together they indicate the color between. This works particularly well for skin and liptones. Hair and eyes are generally multicolored, so either choose a color that matches their general impression or choose the several shades that make up their total color. Remember to match your hair color, not the tone of your latest tint.

The directions for making a Color Key are important. Follow them exactly. This tool will be your inseparable companion wherever you go. I'm never without my Color Key, and I carry one for each member of my family.

Complete directions follow:

— MAKING A COLOR KEY —

1. Cut a ⅝″ x 3″ segment from light cardboard. (Index cards work well for this purpose.)

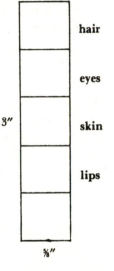

2. Locate a swatch of paper or fabric the color of your hair. (The color plates in the center of this book are the first place to look.) Cut-out any squares that are similar to your hair color. With a mirror and good light, carefully check the assembled colors against your hair. Select the one or two that are closest to your hair color. By selecting two, one on either side of the color you're seeking, you'll have it bracketed. Later, when you find the *exact* shade, you can switch samples.

If your hair has many colors in it, select more than one color to represent your hair.

Be sure to match your own hair color and not the color you've dyed, frosted, bleached or tinted it. Yes, even if your hair is naturally white or salt and pepper. If you haven't seen your own hair color in years and can't match the roots, match the natural color of your eyebrows. They will be similar to your hair color. Don't bypass step two and snip a hank of hair.

You need your color sample to be in a different substance for objectivity.

3. Cut your hair color sample into a ⅝″ square, if it isn't already. With more than one sample, use several narrow strips to make a composite that is ⅝″ square, stacked like a torte. Vary the width of the strips in proportion to amount of color; for instance, a wider dark strip and a narrow band of white for hair that is just turning.

If selecting your exact hair color proves an impossible task due to your inability to "see" fine differences in color, don't despair. Your perception will grow tremendously as you work with color. You can also ask for help from someone with artistic ability and color sensitivity. It will be much easier for them and they may enjoy the exercise. Ask a perceptive friend to check your selection. You want an accurate sample, and additional input can improve your accuracy.

4. Glue your hair-color-sample across one end of the cardboard strip. Rubber cement glues well, for excess glue easily rubs away, and any color can be stripped off when you're able to replace it with a better example. Put a thin coating of cement on the strip, a thin coating on the back of your color sample; wait until they dry; then join the two.

5. Now find the exact color or colors in the iris of your eyes. If your eyes don't match, include both sets of colors. Most eye colors are on the enclosed Color Plates.

6. Once again, cut the color or group of colors into a ⅝″ square and glue the square immediately below your hair sample. Make the two squares touch.

7. Now you're seeking the color of your skin, and one of the Color Plates has a wide selection of skintones. Cut-out the squares most similar to your inside wrist, and check these colors against your face. If you're very tan, match them to a lighter area of your body. Color experts explain that tanning is a change in the skin's value (darkness or lightness), not its hue (color).

If you can't find your exact skin color, once again use two colors which closely bracket it. Keep looking for skintone fabrics, paint chips or clippings-from-magazines. Eventually you'll find that elusive shade.

8. Cut your skintone sample or samples into a single ⅜″ square. Rubber-cement it directly below your eye color.

9. Now, roll your bottom lip down and look at the color on the inside. *This* is the shade that appears in your cheeks when you've just finished two sets of tennis or when you blush. It's also your color-family for lipstick and blusher—the red that is most intimately yours. Find it among the enclosed reds. Cut a ⅜″ square of this color and glue it directly below your skin color.

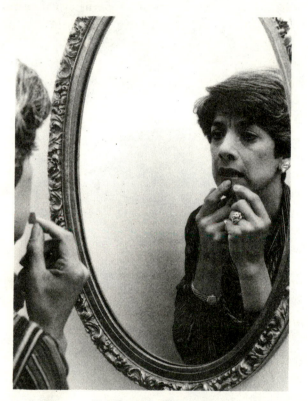

T-3 checking lip color

10. If some of your selections aren't quite perfect, keep searching, but paste-down your best alternates until you find better. Strip-off any nearly-right squares when you have better matches with which to replace them.

11. When satisfied that you've captured your colors, write your name, address and phone number on the back of the strip. You've invested time, cut-up a book and still haven't had time to benefit from your labors. Keep it safe in a plastic cover; *don't lose it.*

12. Save the squares that lost-out by slipping them into an envelope and marking it "colors." This way you can include them when you're selecting colors to wear.

Look at your new Color Key. Isn't it beautiful? The four colors work together to make a blend that is unique and perfect. It's *your* coloring—beautiful without cosmetic aids—key to looking fabulous.

In the next chapter you'll use your new Color Key to select the 200-plus colors that are super on YOU and also to clinch just what Type you are. Make a Color Key, if you haven't, then hurry on ahead.

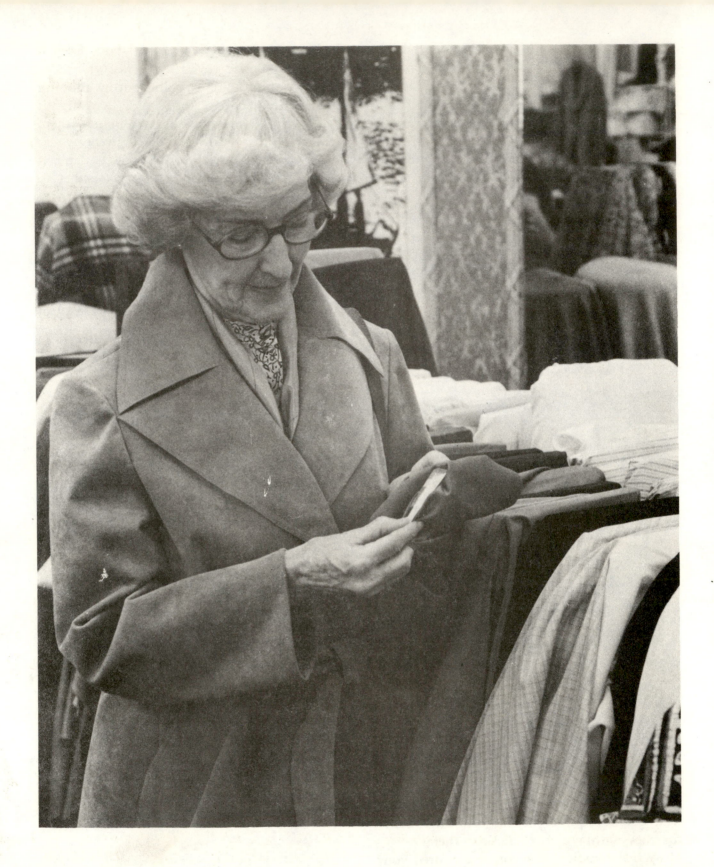

T-2 color shopping fabric with a personal color key

5

Your Colors

With Color Key in hand you're doubtless eager to learn what colors to wear and what harmony you are. That's wonderful, but before you cut the *colors-which-make-you-look-superb* from the Color Plates in the next few pages you'll need to know what to look for and how to find it.

The criteria for *Your Becoming Colors* is that each must enhance every one of the four color squares on your Color Key. Each must make your hair come-alive, your eye color brighten, your skin look yummy and your lip-tone super. Tall order? Yes, indeed, but not as difficult as you may think. Approximately 200 Becoming Colors await your discovery. Each person has that many "great" colors, and each person's are different.

Some colors will enhance your hair, eyes and lips, but dull your skin. Don't be tempted by them. They're not for you. Keep looking. A brightener of your skin that drabs your hair is just as bad. Begin your search for Becoming Colors in the blues, blue-greens, and greens. These hues naturally complement skintone, being across the color-wheel from them. They are, also, very exciting and the easiest to identify as becoming. Check every imaginable blue and green and combination with your Color Key until you find a Becoming one. Look in the dark shades, the light tints, the midranges. Look for all degrees of intensity, from the dullest to the brightest. Remember, to be perfect a color must be beautiful with all *four* sections of your Color Key.

Cut out every color that passes your test.

When you find a blue or green that meets your criteria look at it carefully. It's your entree to all the other wonderful colors you'll wear. Is it bright or grayed? Light or dark? All your Becoming Colors will be similar to this in intensity (being equally bright or muted). You'll find your colors varying in hue enough to almost encircle the color wheel, but they'll retain a common brightness.

Most of your colors will be light or dark or midrange. Find as many as you can. Look for "your" yellows, greens, blues, lavenders, reds and oranges. Next, look for neutrals such as whites, grays, blacks, browns and the non-bright reds, greens, blues and purples. Look for pastels. Can you wear them?

Whatever your type, the darker the shades of your Color Key the darker your Becoming Colors will be. The lighter your coloring, the more likely lighter colors will look best. With high contrast (very light and very dark squares) your colors will be bright. With little contrast you'll select less-brilliant, more-blended tones. Check colors as similar to your own as possible, only hue varying. Discover as many of those 200-plus colors as you can.

See if you can find at least one perfect selection from each color family. You'll unearth a goldmine in some of them.

Your 200 Becoming Colors won't be discovered in one book, one season, or one year; but in a lifetime of looking you'll find more than 200.

A surprising bonus comes with your colors. EACH HARMONIZES WITH EVERY OTHER! Your color combinations can be way-out yet amazingly successful. A small wardrobe will look impressive and you'll reap raves.

Arrange your Becoming Color squares by family, similar tones together. Glue your squares to index cards which have been cut to fit clear-plastic-photo-display leaves in your billfold. Or purchase a separate photo case for your Color Key and Becoming Color Collection. Later, when you shop, you'll look for clothes in these colors plus any other colors which light-up your Color Key.

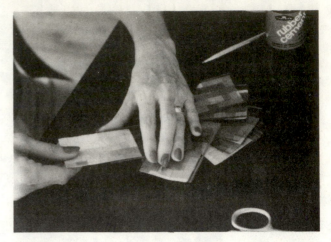

3. **PERSONAL COLOR COLLECTION and COLOR KEY—** completed.

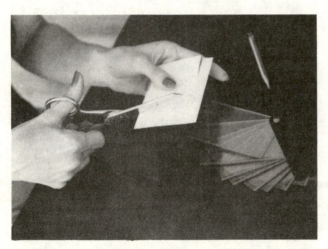

1. **Cutting card to fit protective case.**

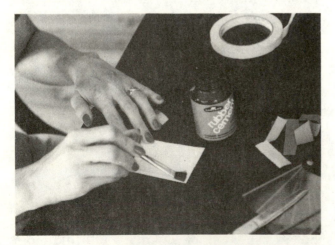

2. **Applying rubber cement to card and to backs of squares. For fabric samples, lay fabric on masking tape, cut to size. Apply glue to the back of tape, let dry, mount as if paper.**

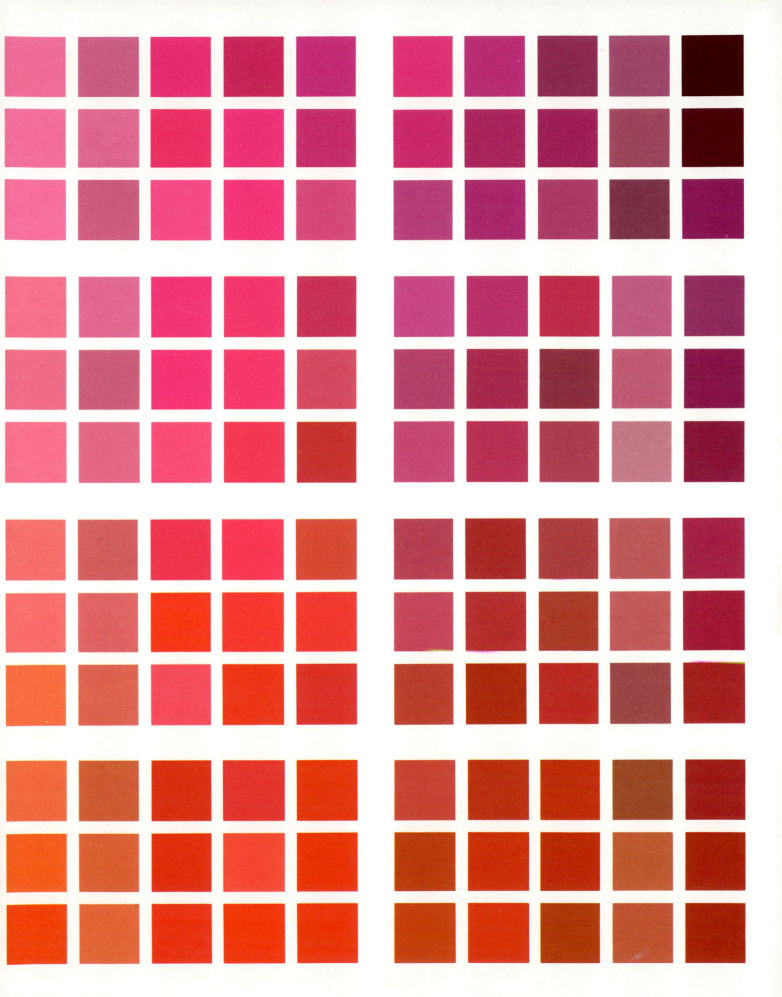

Color Chart A

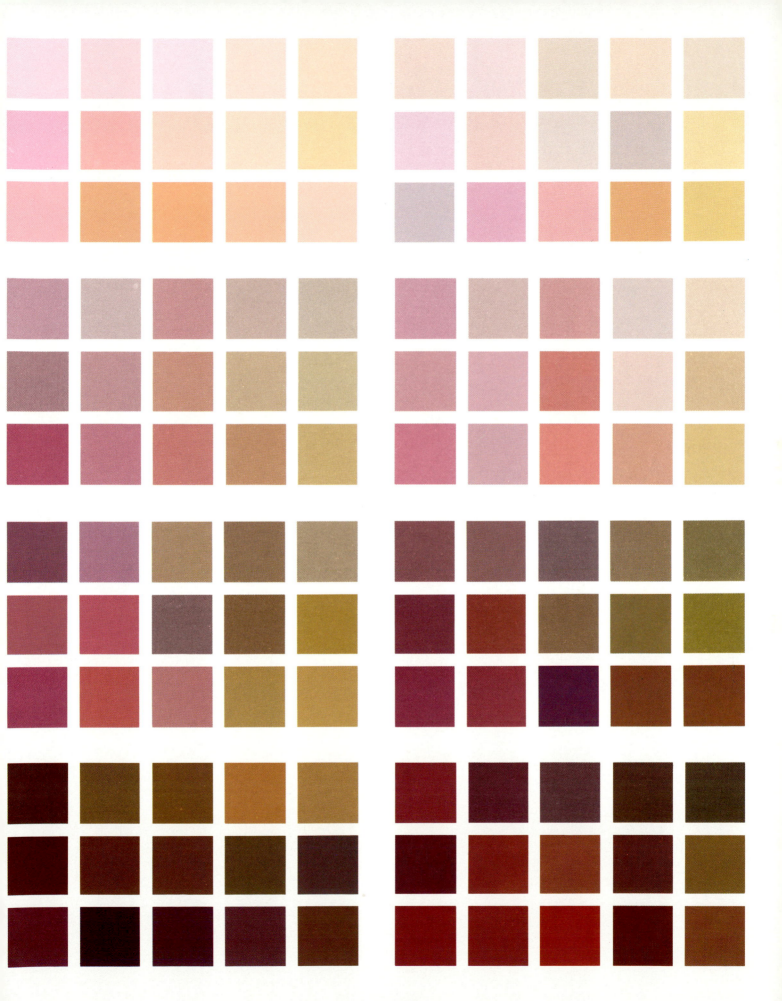

Color Chart B

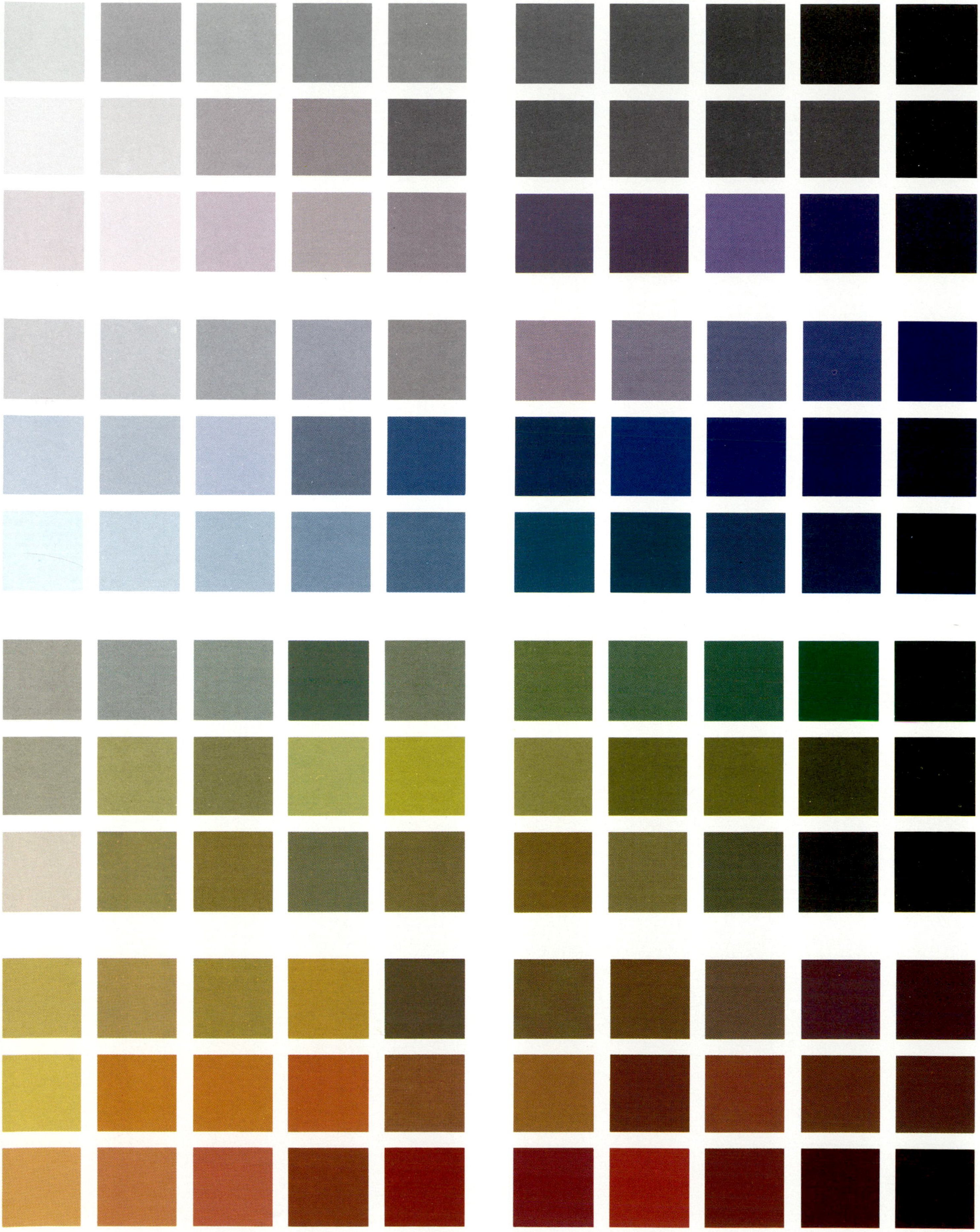

Color Chart C

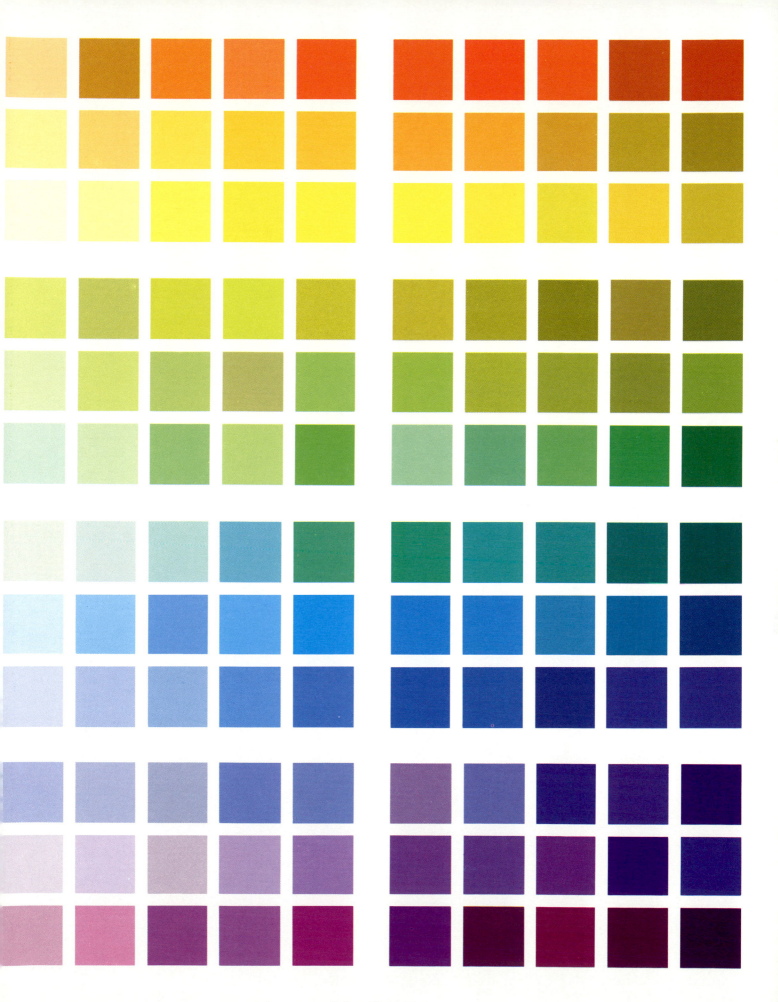

Color Chart D

The ability to perceive which color becomes one and which doesn't is both a gift and a learned skill. You can increase your perception almost immediately by "looking" for subtle differences in color. Don't worry if you have to lean on a friend for a time. Like dancing or playing the clarinet, the ability to recognize fine distinctions comes with practice. Don't give up. After ten years I'm still surprised by the subtleties which once seemed invisible. My abilties slowly and continually develop.

How has the Color Key and your Becoming Color Collection helped you decide which type you are? Again, underline the words in each of the following sections which describe either the colors on your Color Key or those in your Becoming Color Collection. Don't be tempted to underline a color you adore, just because you adore it. Play fair to yourself and underline only those *perfect for you*.

T-1 CHECKLIST F

My colors are: clear, clean, bright.
They include: cool grays, clear grays, blacks, creams, beiges, coffees, medium browns, dark browns, navy blues, lemons, limes, kellys, turquoises, aquas, blueberries, raspberry sherbets, grapes, violets, lilacs, lavenders, roses, strawberries, tomatoes, melons, salmons, peaches, orange sherbets, and tangerines.

Number underlined in T-1 CHECKLIST F
_____.

T-2 CHECKLIST F

My colors are: soft, grayed, blended.
They include: creamy off-whites, grayed beiges, grayed and pinkish browns, clear and blued grays, blacks, dull navys, soft yellows, soft greens, grayed greens, grayed blue-greens, gentle blues, soft purples, lavenders, mauves, delicate blue-reds, soft reds, roses, pinks and peachtones.

Number underlined in T-2 CHECKLIST F
_____.

T-3 CHECKLIST F

My colors are: warm, rich, earthy.
They include: warm grays, blacks, all the browns, coppers, rusts, brownish reds, reddish purples, burgundies, purples, teals, olives, avocados, acid greens, sages, celerys, golds, golden yellows, and pumpkins.

Number underlined in T-3 CHECKLIST F
_____.

T-4 CHECKLIST F

My colors are: brilliant, contrasting, clear.
They include: all the whites, all the blacks, clear grays, bluish grays, brilliant yellows, shocking oranges, scarlets, fuschias, cerises, red-purples, royal purples, bright royal blues, peacock blues, bright aquas, emerald greens, silver and cool bright pastels.

Number underlined in T-4 CHECKLIST F
_____.

The long checklists are over and I imagine you have decided on your Type. Have you found, as I have, that personality, appearance and coloring are matched in each individual? Perhaps you're confused and still don't know which Type you are. In that case, let's head for your Personal Score Card and final answers.

Complete the following record by turning back to each of your test scores. Record those scores on this page in the appropriate sections.

Checklist A's results are on pages 16, 17, 19 and 20.
Checklist B's results are on page 21.
Checklist C's results are on page 21.
Checklist D's results are on pages 24 and 25.
Checklist E's results are on pages 24 and 25.
Checklist F's results are on page 41.

Directions: Transfer results from tests to appropriate columns. With Checklist C, if *introvert* is checked, place five points under Type Two and five under Type Four on line C. If *extrovert* is checked, put five points under Type One and five under Type Three, same line. With Checklist F, multiply your numbers by 10 and record in the appropriate boxes.

_____ 's PERSONAL SCORE CARD

CHECKLIST	Type One	Type Two	Type Three	Type Four
A	22	24	16	33
B	5	4	6	9
C				
D				
E				
F				
TOTALS				

Are your numbers predominately in one division, with some in each of the others? You're okay. You're okay even if your numbers split evenly across all four divisions, although this is rare. Which column has the most points? *That indicates your Type!* With a tie, or two columns with nearly identical totals, note the color test, Checklist F. Consider the highest score on Checklist F the winner. Colors that are right on you will always indicate your Type . . . they break ties.

Circle the highest total. Your Type heads that column. Now you know which Type you are, and you need that information, for the following suggestions and instructions will be given by Type. Read what *each* Type wears. You'll learn faster that way.

What Do You Choose?

6
Wonderland

Musical background for our journey through Type One's territory might well be Tchaikovsky's "Nutcracker Suite." Dwell lightly on dancing dandelions, tutued hippos, darting butterflies, perky pansies, bumbling mushrooms, and all the Disney characters, sans villians, from Peter Pan to Herbie to Sleeping Beauty. Color your musings with bright paints or gentle pastels. Round the shapes. Smooth the textures. Now you have it . . . a collage of Type One illustrations.

But, how do you use imagery? You keep it in mind, for nothing you choose for your person, if you're a Type One, must violate the spirit of *Wonderland*.

To be practical . . .

T-1s number in the millions yet no two are alike. They have differing lifestyles, bodies, and budgets. Additionally, fashion items change yearly. How can I recommend a navy flannel blazer with shiny brass buttons? I can't, even though that blazer would work for most. I have to give guidelines instead of answers.

Pencil and paper time again!

Arrange those Type Ones you know in order from largest and darkest to smallest and fairest. At the top of your list may be Karen or Greg, slim, dark haired, maybe dark eyed, with dramatic enthusiasm. Next may come Susan or Eric, square shouldered, straightforward, with a no-nonsense attitude. Somewhere in the middle would be Becky or John, medium contrast, lively sports enthusiasts

who adore the outdoors. Then we'd have Carol or Cliff, classic, cool, with a tinge of royalty in their outlook and bearing. Near the bottom of your list would be the small, fair, quiet Lisa or Larry, possible pixies or innocents.

Where do *you* fit on the list? Near the top? Near the bottom? Can you shoehorn yourself into the T-1 list or are you one of the other types?

I'll be listing Type One colors, fabrics, furs, fabric designs, detailing, clothing, and accessories in descending lists, approximately comparable to the list you prepared of people, when I can. Not all objects or finishes can be listed that way, unfortunately.

While one clothing idea may look superior on a majority of T-1s, another enhances only a few. Try *everything* to learn which items work for you.

As you test this theory you'll find Type Ones with the most contrast (dark and light) push toward Type Four clothing yet stop short of T-4s total simplicity. Such a T-1 might wear a black and white floral print with either black or white strongly dominating. Type Four *never* wears floral.

Those with the least contrast (paler people) approach Type Two's soft clothing yet with gentle crispness, brightness or motion. Such a T-1 would choose slightly crisp lace or delicate, swinging earrings.

Type Ones who share a strong secondary with Type Three may borrow T-3 themes, but

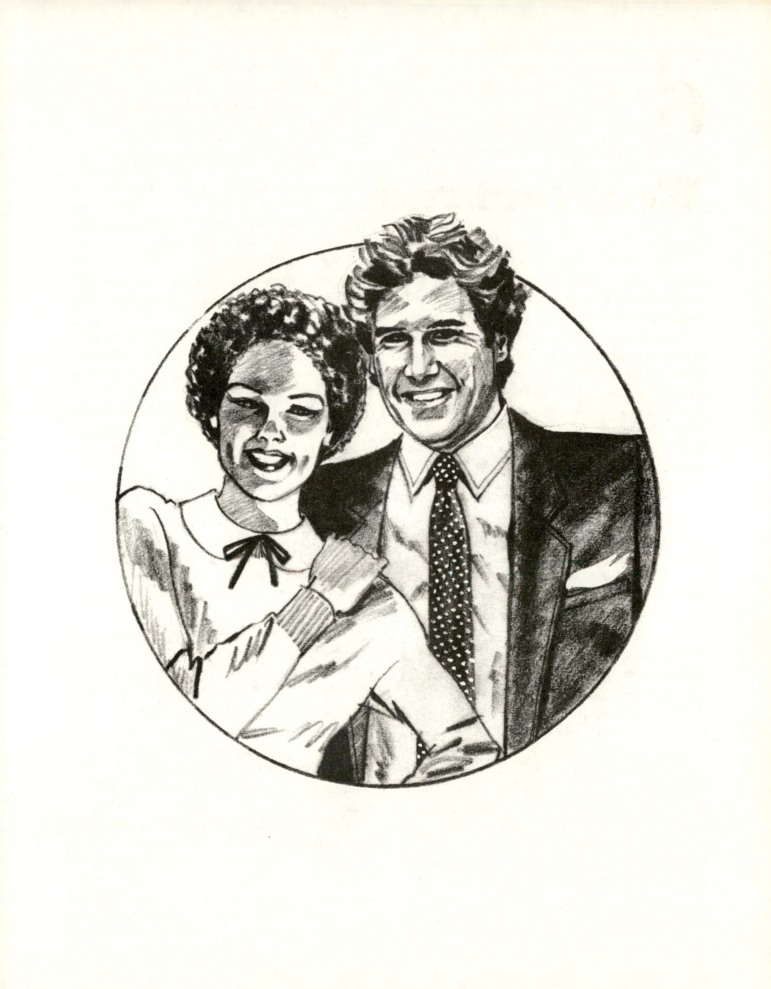

with coolness and polish. This kind of T-1 may choose a smooth, almost-invisible plaid for suiting. T-3s often wear plaids.

— COLORS —

Type One colors are clear, bright, fresh, appealing. They may be saturated with sunlight, warm or cool, water-washed or opaque, delicate or deep. They are eye catching, clean and perky as the flowers of spring, airy as a butterfly.

Those T-1s with darker hair and eyes will choose full-strength brights plus darks and lights. T-1s with paler hair and eyes will choose the light pastels with no blacks or dark tones. In-betweens will choose diffused brights or sherbet colors with some lights and darks. Your colors are the exact ones you found in chapter 5, those which make you sparkle.

T-1s use brights with bright. They wear red with purple, green with blue; or yellow, red and purple in the same outfit. Restraint is found only in proportion . . . one color must dominate and others be in uneven amounts.

T-1s add brights to their neutrals. Too bubbly to be verbally quiet, they add colorful ties, shirts, blouses, scarves, ascots or jewelry to their more sober outfits.

T-1s avoid dim, dusky, murky, gloomy, somber, mysterious and oppressive colors.

— FABRICS —

The following fabrics look exciting on Type Ones, reinforcing personalities, bone structure and coloring:

felt, velveteen, wool jersey, cotton and wool flannel, cotton twill and ottoman, linen, shantung, sharkskin, polyester and wool gabardine, duck, poplin, lightweight canvas, shiny polyurethane, oiled taffeta, taffeta, crisp lace, tie silk, smooth/crisp knits, pointelle, fine cable and popcorn stitches, fine wale corduroy, kettlecloth, pique, oxford, trigger, polished cotton, denim, broadcloth, fine seersucker, ribcord, chambray, percale, smooth muslin, brushed nylon, terry,

calico, gingham, chintz, voile, organdy, organza, crepe georgette, dotted Swiss, eyelet, net and batiste.

Leathers and furs cover like fabrics. Let's consider them next.

— LEATHERS AND FURS —

Alas, the saddest news, T-1s weren't designed to trail sable . . . they're much too young visually. Rare or lush skins belong on their more sophisticated friends.

But what furs *can* they wear? Or is that the wrong question? Shouldn't we ask how they can best wear fur to enhance their youthfulness? That's better!

Any treatment that is lighthearted is for Type One. Think fun furs . . . those fabulous fakes. Think of battle jackets, ski parkas or trench coats lined in fur, trimmed with fur or even made of fur . . . but fur that doesn't take itself seriously. Think of a curly lamb shrug, a squirrel jacket, or a reversed sheepskin parka with colorful embroidery. Think of seal, weasel and dyed rabbit used like fabric. Think smooth, lightweight calf, suede and patent leather.

The lightest colors and gayest treatments belong to those T-1s who are fair. Their darker brothers and sisters look for simpler, more classic lines, but lines holding a hint of tongue-in-cheek.

To be avoided: the great cats, the monied look!

— FABRIC DESIGNS —

Knowing which fabrics and furs work for each harmony is a great help, but fabric isn't always plain. It also comes printed, flocked or striped. How do you know if a print will contribute a plus or a minus to your look? These enhance T-1s:

tartan plaid, tattersall, racing and candy stripes, nautical and Tyrolean themes; *geometrics:* check, star, coin and polka dots, circle, equilateral triangle, bubble and teardrop, but *not paisley,* scattered design as opposed to static, all flowers except the exotic, patchwork, cottage and border prints, flocking, lace, monogram, tennis racket, lock and key, heart, butterfly, owl, turtle, strawberry and mushroom.

Have the preceeding cute designs turned you off? Sorry. I'm a T-1 yet I rarely wear floral and never choose owls and turtles. I *do* have a gold butterfly for my ascot and a silver heart for my lapel. You might enjoy a tennis racket design on a non-business tie.

Don't forget to relate a design's scale to your size, it's contrast (darkness or lightness) to your own contrast, and it's colors to those becoming to you.

Avoid prints with chalk-white backgrounds if chalk-white is not one of your colors. Mid-range brights and neutrals were made for T-1s . . . good luck in finding them.

Check all the colors in a multi-colored print. Don't buy a print having more than one non-good color, nor having that one color in more than a minor amount.

Six Criteria for a Good Print
1. Interesting shapes and motifs, arranged rhythmically
2. Harmony of several motifs by some unity in size or shape
3. Pleasing variety
4. Interesting background spaces
5. Lights and darks lying on one surface, not leaping at you.
6. The designer's statement clearly expressed

— GARMENT DETAILING —

What design details belong to Type One? They include the following, but round or curving is the key to lapels, pockets, necklines, buttons, buckles and seams.

Necklines: halter, bowed, boatneck, crew, keyhole, sweetheart, gathered, scoop, jewelry and round. **Collars:** shirt, button-down, shirtband, sailor, petal, Peter Pan, crystal pleats, ruffles and Pierrot. **Sleeves:** sleeveless, capped, puffed, angel, three-quarter and long. **Hems:** shirt-tail, hand-kerchief, picot, crocheted, scalloped, flared, fluted and lettuce. **Also:** strapless, spaghetti straps, peplums, midriff-tied, accordian and umbrella pleats, tucking, smocking, gathers, yokes, bib fronts, drawstring ruffles, crinolines, contrast stitching and trims, piping, braids, rick-rack, trapunto, ribbon (satin and gros-grain), flowered and striped braids, ruffles, scallops, nautical and peasant detailing, oversize zippers, rows of buttons, fun grommets, lacings, applique, openwork, lace, ribbon-laced eyelet, heart-shaped pockets, bows and embroidery.

Avoid: the exotic and the elegant!

— TYPES OF CLOTHING —

Names and styles change, one's figure limits choices, and personal taste dictates the inclusion/exclusion of apparel items. You won't like and can't wear *all* the following, but each supports T-1's uniqueness.

Coats: trench, balmacaan, wrap, princess-style, polo, pea and rain slicker. **Jackets:** nylon windbreaker, aviator, Eisenhower, jean, pea, Spencer, ski parka, blazer and bolero, jogging warm-up, quilted vest and triangular stole. **Shirts:** turtleneck, polo, tee, peasant and western, ruffled, tucked, bowed and yoked. **Dresses:** shirt, peasant, tee, dressmaker and sailor. **Also:** jumpsuits, jumpers, pinafores, smocks, elasticized bodices and waists, terry and quilted robes, baby doll pajamas. **Jeans:** western, modified, cigarette, hip-hugger and bell-bottom. **Pants:** slacks, drawstring, warm-up, high-rise, culotte, tennis shorts, boxer, gym, tap and short-shorts, trunks, bikinis for those with the figure, or boy-leg swimsuits. **Skirts:** kilts, flared, wrapped, gathered, multi-pleated, multi-tiered, dirndl, straight and A-line.

— ACCESSORIES —

Perfectly-chosen accessories finish your look and add impact, but they need to be of good quality and reinforce *you*. Choose from the following:

Headgear: caps—baseball, sports car, sailor, Ali McGraw, watch and tam, tennis visor, kerchief tied peasant-style; hats—beret, Breton, sailor, southwester, cowboy, derby, dome, perforated straw, bonnet and halo; trimmings—ribbon, lace, flower and veil, plus fantasy like Robinhood's feathered chapeau.

Scarves and Ties: light-weight, smooth-surfaced, crisp fabrics in bright or neutral solids, or prints which follow the guidelines under Fabric Designs, page 47; for business—solids, diagonal stripes, polka dots, or regularly spaced all-over patterns of tiny objects—nothing else . . . except bow ties when in fashion.

Watches: round and shiny of silver, stainless or gold. Round face. Avoid jewels and ornateness. For casual wear, a colored face, dive watch, sport band, plastic case or Mickey Mouse compliments the young or young-in-heart.

Belts: width varies with fashion, but T-1s choose smooth leather with shiny, rounded buckles for business. Leather thongs, shiny patent, straw, linen, ribbon and elastic add variety for dress and play.

Bags and Wallets: smooth leather in a neutral color is best for business . . . dark brown secretary-type wallet for the breast pocket is preferred for men as is a dark-brown attache case, expensive, with lock (in lieu of a purse for women). Also, in season, patent, canvas, wicker, straw and plastic with bright, rounded, metal trim or contrast stitching. Think of saddle bags, totes, hobos, clutches, envelopes, pouches and duffles.

Shoes: young styles, smooth materials, rounded details, simplicity. Boots—cowboy, engineer's, and "city" in black, navy, brown, butterscotch or maroon. Shoes—pumps, spectators, Mary Janes, baby dolls, T-straps, ankle straps, slides, yo-yos, espadrilles, loafers, tennies, strappy sandals and pom-pomed mules, slides, slip-ons. Details—moccasin toes, stacked heels, contrast stitching and trim, perforations and round, shiny buckles.

Jewelry: corporate males wear only a wedding band . . . no tie tacks, cufflinks or school rings. Corporate females choose highly polished round earrings and a simple, expensive-looking chain or lapel pin in gold or silver. After hours or in other jobs, the bright and amusing are choices: smooth round beads, creamy pearls, thin gold or silver chains, airy rings of gold loops or flowers or butterflies, heart-shaped silver pin or key-chain ornament, paperclip-links sterling bracelet, enamel on silver, porcelain or glass flowers, straw flowers, fabric flowers on silken cords, charm bracelets, flower-painted wooden bangles, all the fruit/animal/geometric designs turned into 3-D jewelry. Choose bright colors where possible. *Avoid chalk white, angular pieces and those with antiquing or roughness.*

Gloves and Fans: when fashionable. Choose youngster's mittens, driving gloves, or elegant kidskin. Fans may be of paper, feathers or straw. Muffs add feminine fun.

Shopping tricks will be given in later chapters, but don't be tempted to skip the next 3 chapters, whatever your type. You need to thoroughly understand *each* of the four Types in order to avoid selection errors. *Learning what's wrong for you is almost as good as learning what's right!*

7

Camelot

Gear down to the 13th Century landscape, the legends of Camelot, the romantic age for which Type Twos were fashioned.

Enjoy the richness of tapestry and banner, silk and velvet, hooded fur, sweeping gown, pearls and filligree, or his slashed doublet, tunic, silken hose, sword, cape and gracefully plumed hat.

Glimpse movement through a narrow window. Gallant knight in shining armor, milady's favor upon his sleeve, controls his steed, while she, soft with furs, tosses him a single flower.

Romantic clothing from past eras flatter T-2s and should be first choices for costume parties, but equally becoming selections are available for daily wear.

Before we discuss clothing choices, let's look at the differences within the family of Twos.

As we did with Type Ones, arrange T-2s into descending order from largest and darkest to smallest and fairest.

The list would be topped with Mona and Edward who're tall, slightly angular, dark-haired and dark-eyed with pale, elongated faces. Their high contrast (difference in darkness and lightness) indicates a need for colors with depth and even a measure of brightness. On well-proportioned bodies, high fashion clothes can look marvelous, but T-2s are never flamboyant. They strive for sophisticated elegance and refined drama.

Grace and Claude have more classic features and average height. You may think of them as poised and gracious, almost regal. Patricians, they choose highly refined, luxurious fabrics, graceful lines and colors which flow together—always the cultured look.

Rose and Terrance are sturdier with a somewhat athletic build. Naturally casual, they wear less formal clothing, but their selections are simple, well-cut designs of genuine worth. They choose brown suede instead of burgundy velvet.

Romantic epitomizes Melanie and Bryan. Their eyes are large and warm, lips curving . . . she the Southern belle, he the Cavalier. They're willowy and graceful. Red is often their favorite color and luxurious fabrics their clothing forte.

Smallest and fairest of T-2s are Violet and Lance with their youthful faces, lighter skin and hair, more delicate bone structure and Alice-in-Wonderland eyes. Humor and dash is checked by gentleness, and their wardrobes hold spirited touches, the new or the quaintly picturesque.

You fail to fit these descriptions? Don't worry. With millions of people in each category, one page of sketches may easily miss you. Keep working with T-2 ideas and your special look will emerge . . . if you're in this harmony. You can try the clothes of T-2s to see how, or if, they suit; but first you'll need to understand how Type Two uses color.

— COLORS —

Type Two colors are soft, shadowy, blended. Although brightness is muted, your shades glow with inner life as do fine jewels. No harsh surprises here, please.

Rose or blue tones may tint all your colors. Values may be dark or light, intensity muted or nearly bright. Look for iridescent or pearlized forms, misty tints or heathery blends. T-2 colors are listed on page 41, but if there is ever a question of buying the red or the any-other-color item, choose the red. It emphasizes your romantic nature.

T-2s use gradations of the same color, a monochromatic color scheme—each tone blending into the next.

T-2s use closely related colors, the analogous color scheme—blue used with lavender, red with deep pink or red-purple.

T-2s avoid contrast, dark and light used together. They choose all-dark, all-light, or all mid-range values.

T-2s avoid muddy, clear, brilliant or heavy colors and combinations like red, white and blue.

— FABRICS —

The following fabrics enhance Type Two's sensitive features and gentle nature:

suede, Ultrasuede, fine wool flannel, wool crepe, cashmere, heathery wools, mohair, wool challis, wool jersey, velvet, panné velvet, velveteen, velour, brushed denim, no-wale corduroy, damask, floral jacquard, tapestry, linen, soft knits, matte jersey, satin remarque, satin, delusterized satin, moiré, watered taffeta, crepe de chine, crepe georgette, Nyesta, Qiana, silk marquisette, hand-painted silk, handkerchief linen, voile, lawn, fluid polyester, cire, soft lace, cobweb lace, chiffon, shadow-striped chiffon, mousseline and charmeuse.

— LEATHERS AND FURS —

Whereas Type One looks for fun furs, Type Two seeks refined pelts. T-2 glows in luxurious:

chinchilla, summer ermine, soft brown or taupe mink, blue fox, golden or dark Russian sable, moiré, caracul and soft-toned broadtail lamb, Russian squirrel, opossum, fisher and mole. Enhancing styles include: hood, cloche, bonnet, bag, cape, stole, collar, boa, jacket and coat—both street and floor lengths. Leather should be butter-soft and smooth—high-quality calf, suede and kidskin.

Avoid patterned fur, stark white, contrasting trim, young styles or anything which looks inexpensive.

Consider lining a cloth coat with fur . . . perhaps a fur lining that could be zipped alternately into a garnet velvet evening coat, a taupe moiré raincoat, and a grey suede topcoat. A male of this harmony should consider a fur hat with cloth coat, or fur collar and lining for his traditional trenchcoat.

— FABRIC DESIGNS —

"Better a solid than a print that sabotages," could be Type Two's motto, for most prints prove overpowering. Designs that don't overpower include: delicate embossing, tone-on-tone sheers, flowing S lines, atmospheric prints, indistinct swirls of color, sunlight filtering through shade, the delicacy of a Renoir, cascading flowers like languid wisteria, nodding fuschia and full-blown roses. All designs have elegance, softness and a blended quality.

Avoid prints with contrast, brilliance or unbecoming colors.

Avoid prints which are bold, ordinary or out-of-scale with your body.

— GARMENT DETAILING —

An *oval* reinforces the essence of a T-2, so look for the ovalized lapel, neckline, button,

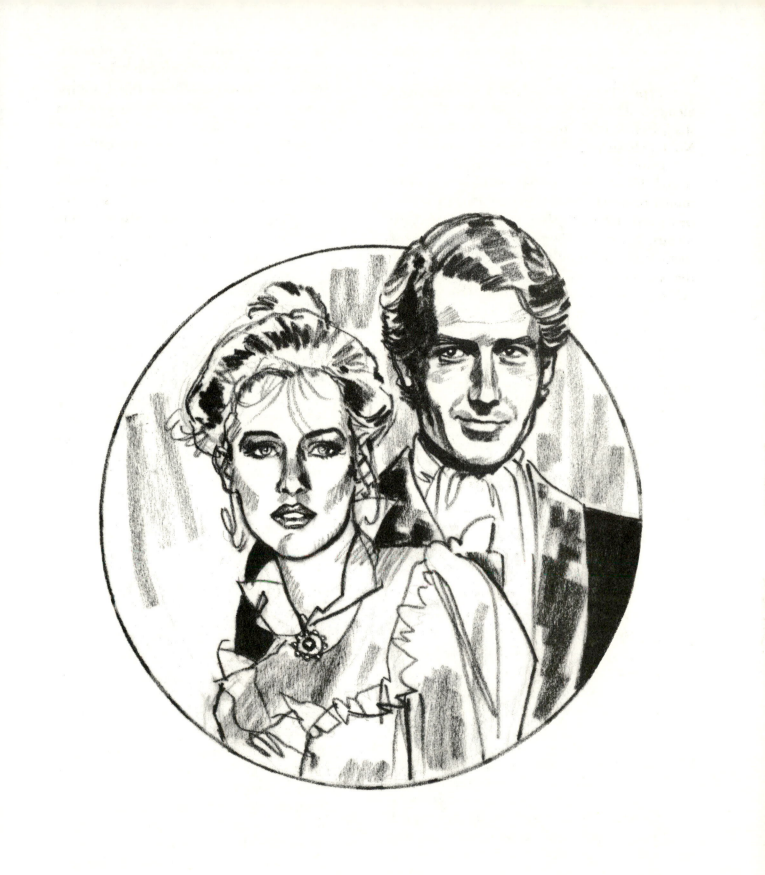

buckle and seaming. The following also contribute positively:

Necklines: a covered look (no tops open to the navel)—oval, curved, gathered, draped, bateau, cowl, jewelry, turtle, limply ruffled/flounced/bowed, off-the-shoulder or face-framing effects, all rounded rather than angular. **Collars:** oval, vertical rather than horizontal effects, bertha, shawl, curved, ascot, Pierrot, hood, flounced, lace-inset. **Sleeves:** puffed, poet, angel, bell, butterfly, three-quarter, long, set-in, dolman, batwing, deep cuffed, maribou trimmed or lace cuffed.

Hems: handkerchief, picot, flared, fagotted, fluted, godeted. **Also:** floating panels, streamers, draped/flared/gathered backs, flowing or slim lines, sashes, empire waists, tucking, gathers, ribbon (satin and velvet are best), garlands, ostrich feathers, rows of tiny buttons, lacings (if delicate), soft lace and embroidery.

Avoid the exotic and the ordinary.

— TYPES OF CLOTHING —

A wardrobe of romantically-elegant styles is your goal, so think ensemble dressing. Coordinate separates into costumes, choosing from the following:

Capes: all lengths **Coats:** cashmere, mohair, ultra-suede, velvet or silk—in wrap, princess, back-belted or shawl-collared styles. Fur collars are perfect. **Jackets:** cut-velvet or velvet smoking styles, Nehru collars, English-cut, hacking style, velvet or fur collars, soft suede. **Suits:** luxurious fabric, romantic cut, jackets and skirt/pants of same or similar color. Emphasize the vertical with slash pockets (not patch) and vertical seaming. **Stoles:** silky, frothy, fluff, feathers or fur. **Shirts:** turtleneck, cowl, classic, tucked, soft bow, full sleeve, artist's smock, tunic. **Dresses:** princess-line, lace-trimmed dressmaker, cowled sweater, 2-piece knit, elegant peasant, empire, long-waisted. **Also:**

fine-fabric jumpsuits, vertical jumpers, knit vests, velvet/silk/chiffon robes, negligees, peignoirs, lace-lavished nightgowns, elegant camisoles and teddys. **Jeans:** straight-legged velvet, velveteen or brushed denim. **Pants:** slacks, high-waist, culotte (especially long), shorts covered by a skirt, draped or skirted swimsuits, maillots. **Skirts:** flared, wrapped, gathered, tiered, paneled, dirndl, A-line and slim.

— ACCESSORIES —

Type One and Three can use odd, kooky or inexpensive accessories, but not Types Two and Four. The latter types have an elegance which demands fine quality. Type Twos choose from the following:

Headgear: fine-wool sports car cap, deer-stalker, homburg, snapbrim, beret, turban, dome, helmet, soft cartwheel, picture, bonnet, hood, snood. Trimming could be fur, lace, veiling, ribbons, streamers or flowers. Picture her hair in a Frenchtwist wrapped with open black veiling and secured with an ear-covering black silk rose. **Scarves and Ties:** lightweight, smooth-surfaced, soft fabrics in your colors, either print or plain. Look for: ascot, cravat, jabot, cashmere or silk muffler, scarf twisted with pearls or delicate chains, long chiffon scarf (ends floating instead of knotted). Ties should contrast little with shirt in color or value. They may be solid, tone-on-tone, pearlized, moiréd—in an all-over or diagonal pattern, watercolor print, or delicate abstract. Choose long rather than bow ties except for formal attire, the string tie on occasion, but *never* the narrow cord with a rough rock slide.

Watches: oval, of brushed silver or gold. Numerals may be either Roman (I, II, II) or Arabic (1, 2, 3) but the watch must look expensive. Since timepieces are basically utilitarian, jeweled cases are not recommended, but tasteful scrollwork or filigree is acceptable.

Belts: soft suede should be a first choice with an oval buckle of suede, brushed silver or gold. Soft calf or kidskin plus self-fabric belts, either buckled or tied are suitable, as are sashes, cummerbunds and cascading ribbons. **Bags and Wallets:** soft or sueded leather is correct for business if in a neutral (maroon, brown, taupe, gray or black). Both secretary wallets and expensive attaches with lock are recommended for all Types. Outside of business, look for oval lines in clutch, pouch, envelope and shoulder bags. Materials should be luxurious . . . tapestry, damask, suede, silk, velvet, ottoman, kid, pearlized, beaded, goldleaf, brushed silver or gold . . . worked flat or gathered. Add a muff purse if ever you can. **Shoes:** elegant styles with simplicity and delicacy, oval toes and detailing, quality materials are a must. Classic for the female may be a closed toe and heel pump in softest taupe suede, a slingback with draped vamp, or a refined dress boot. Her at-home slippers could be simple ballerinas or high-heeled mules with open rose on the toe. His footwear may be a dark dress boot with the feel of glove leather, a patent-leather dancing slipper for evening or the more casual jodphur boot. Beware the heavy or cloddy. **Jewelry:** limited at work to a wedding band, simple earrings, pearls, or a pin of satin-finished gold or silver. T-2s wear exquisite jewelry with a look of age but never crudely-formed antiquities. Look for fanciful engraving on a pocketwatch and use it with chain and fob, glowing cameos, filligreed lavalier, oval locket on narrow velvet ribbon, knotted satin strands, silken cords, clusters of stones instead of solitaires, especially opals, amethysts, garnets, cabochon emeralds, smooth pink coral, pearls, diamonds with pearls, pave or rose-cut diamonds, and other glowing or iridescent jewelry. Be a princess in your strings of pearls, especially those with pink and cream tints, frosted crystal beads, slender gold or silver chains. The silken rose tucked into hair, decolletage, or onto a band at throat or wrist would be lovely.

Avoid: brilliant, rough, crude, square, modern, youthful or noisy pieces, like charm bracelets.

Gloves and Fans: Gloves add polish to T-2s costume, so wear then when fashion allows. Longer gloves bring elegance to an evening gown and in kid or doeskin are immensely flattering. Fans, except the fun versions, were made for T-2s. Own several: feathered, silken, delicately handpainted or carved, and learn to flirt with them. You alone could reverse the trend, for romantic eyes and fans belong together. Male version of the fan might be the slender walking stick.

Each harmony has beautiful, coordinated materials and lines from which to select. Each seems more beautiful than the last, and you may be tempted to steal from another's group because you so love that item. Don't do it! Use another's things in your home, if you *must* have them around, or buy them to give to that other person, but don't wear them. Keep all the attention on YOU.

Type Three's clothes have the most WOW of all. You'll see why in the next chapter.

8

Atlantis

Lush vegetation, exotic animals, powerful warriors and Amazons spell Type Three adventure—but not merely primitive Tarzan style. Citizens of Atlantis aimed for world supremacy and had enough scientific information and military might to obtain it.

The Atlantean populace, apparently similar in appearance to the tallest of American Indians, wore striking furs, hammered gold armor, jeweled headdresses and girdles. They looked like conquerors.

But energy, ambition and knowledge weren't enough. Arrogance and materialism, the very traits Type Threes need most to guard against, brought about the fall of Atlantis.

You T-3s resemble the Atlanteans, so choose strong, earthy, exotic clothing statements. The young, elegant, or ordinary are not for you.

Are all Type Threes Amazons and warriors? No, only a few. Let's look at typical T-3s who range from tallest and darkest to shortest and fairest.

Tall, dark and handsome describes Rita and Jose as do the words angular and fascinating.

Equally tall, but with finer skin and fewer angles, Sheila and Douglas possess a more polished, regal appearance. Their clothing, selected from high fashion or classic lines, always exhibits an unusual touch (ornate medallion? turban?).

Anna and Max are sturdy, broad-shouldered, relaxed. With lighter complexions and more casual attitudes, this pair looks best in either strong, bright colors or earthtones. Well-cut tweed suits, coats or jackets with woven-leather buttons should always be a part of their wardrobes.

Highly decorative describes Desiree and Guy. Long lashes, a straight nose and rich coloring lend each a sensuous beauty. Garment choices of slinky fabrics in low-cut or open front styles often reveal fine figures.

Ginger and Ted are the smallest of this group. They're twinkly-eyed and decidedly spicy in manner as well as in Becoming Colors. What happy gypsies!

— COLORS —

Type Three colors are warm, earthy and rich. They may be bright as a parrot or dull as loam, but each has a touch of black, brown or gold in it. If you've ever mixed paint you know a tiny touch of black or brown turns lemon-yellow, golden. A small amount changes clear-green to avocado, sage, poison or green-with-an-acidic-edge. These mature tones hint of harvest, fall leaves, oxidized metals and furry animals.

The stronger your coloring—the more vivid your colors. The lighter or quieter your coloring—the less vivid.

T-3s use their bright colors in wild combinations.

T-3s use neutrals texturally. Think tweed, herringbone, diagonal ribbing or random slub fabrics.

T-3s avoid clear, crisp colors (especially chalk white and light blue) and combinations like red/white/blue. Leave these for T-1s or T-4s.

Enhance your image of fire, passion, earth with warm colors. Cool colors put out your fire.

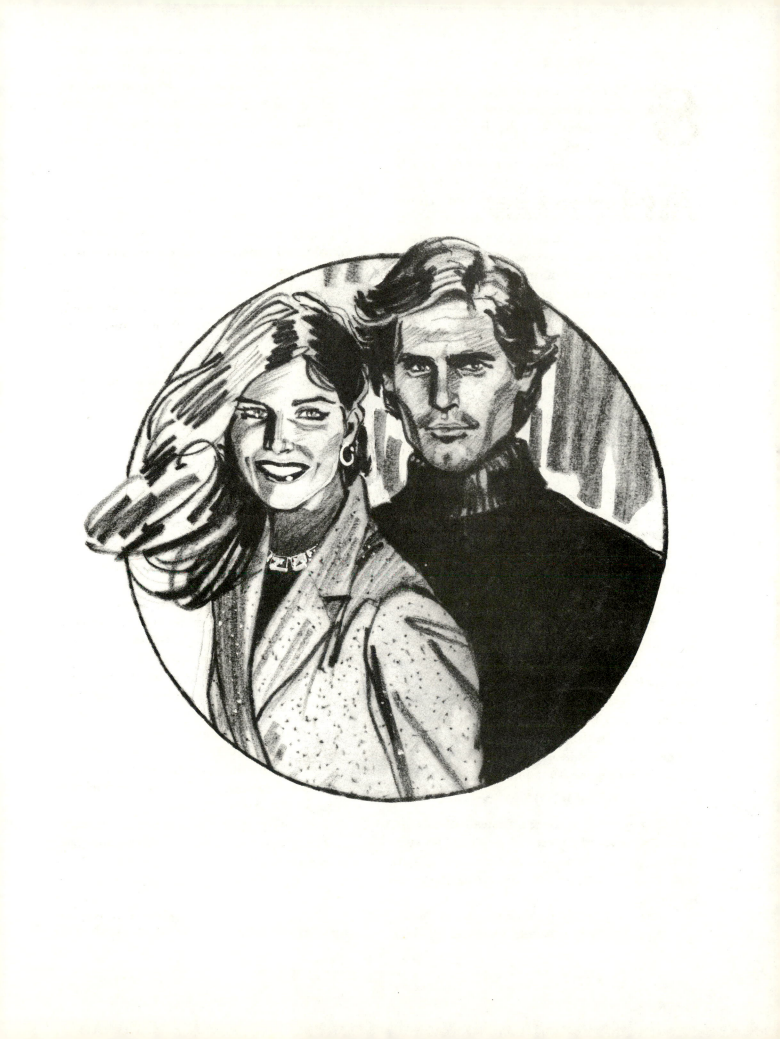

— FABRICS —

Type Three's built-in textural interest demands fabric with surface interest, pattern or tactile excitement; so look for:

raw silk, tweed, rough wool, menswear, herringbone, covert, whipcord, twill, diagonal weaves, camelhair, wide-wale corduroy, slub silk, tie silk, sari cloth, foulard, homespun, slub linen, sisal, pongee, Batik, French or crinkle gauze, Hoya, Honan, madras, plaid, bias warp, fishnet, kettlecloth, muslin, canvas, terry, chenille, bouclé, jacquard, slinky or textured knit, metallic knit, jersey, printed and panné velvet, rich brocade (especially metallic), satin, hammered and crepeback satin, lamé, open knit, see-through sheers, and hand-knit wool.

— LEATHERS AND FURS —

Type Three was born to wear fur . . . all the sensuous or textural skins you can afford. Rare pelts are excitingly patterned, so look for the semblance of jungle cats: ocelot, lynx, jaguar, leopard, tiger. Star in coyote, wolf, red fox, stencil-dyed blue fox, raccoon, skunk, muskrat, beaver, badger, squirrel, otter, opossum, nutria, natural rabbit, Persian lamb, shearling, stonemarten and seal. But be kind to our world and avoid *endangered* species. Their unique colorings and patterns can be stenciled onto other furs or synthetics.

Glamour furs, if you insist on them, look best when worked in stripes, diagonals or chevrons. Think of mink-on-the-bias.

Split cowhide, pigskin, snake, alligator and ostrich belong to you as does rough, fringed suede. Oh for a cold winter!

Avoid safe, ordinary or young furs.

— FABRIC DESIGNS —

Choose a T-3 design instead of single-color material whenever it's possible, because pattern matches the excitement of your skin and hair. Examples of becoming patterns include:

ethnic—Egyptian, African, Aztec, Mexican, Spanish, Indian, Oriental, Malay-sian, Persian, Gypsy; *geometric*—diagonal, zig-zag, argyle or Harlequin, square, rectangle, hexagon, octagon, stripe, plaid, arrow, brick and tile, diagonal quilting; *exotic*—jungle, leopard, lion, zebra, giraffe, snake, dragon, feather, leaf, flame, rattan, bamboo, mosaic, paisley, tapestry; *unusual flora*—chrysanthemum, anthureum, bird-of-paradise, orchid, leaves with angularity and sharpness.

Bizarre and audacious prints belong to you, as do all quietly textured knit and woven goods. *Texture is your key.*

Don't forget . . . relate a design's scale to your size (large patterns on large people, small on small), its contrast (dark or lightness) to your own contrast, and its colors to those becoming to you.

Avoid prints with white backgrounds.

Avoid nursery animals. Your cats are full-grown, not kittens.

— GARMENT DETAILING —

What design details should you seek? Best include the angular, the diagonal, the swift change of direction.

Necklines: open, plunging, or high-yet-revealing, V'd halter, V, turtleneck, boat-neck, side opening, square, rectangular, drawstring, strapless, thong-laced. **Collars:** shirt, deep notch, sharp point, Nehru, mandarin, frog closed, banded. No up-tight looks. **Sleeves:** kimono, Kabuki, dolman, batwing, set-in, sleeveless, one sleeve only, elbow and gun patches. **Hems:** shirttail, standard, fringed, curved as on a sarong, uneven, slit high. **Also:** side closings, wrap styles, sexy peasant looks, midriff-tied, ethnic embroidery, suede lacing and fringe, obi/thong/braided beltings, epaulets, toggles and leather piping.

Aim for irregular and informal balance.

Avoid curving lines, gathers, too-cool, too-mannish. Last item is okay for guys!

— TYPES OF CLOTHING —

With such a wild array of choices, remember to select only the items which reinforce YOU, not all that are listed. A Type Three dissimilar to you will gleefully choose those you cannot.

Coats: military, wrap, dolman-sleeved, trench, balmacaan, duffle, poncho or sweeping cape with a tassel on the hood. **Jackets:** if limited to one, make it a TWEED, but seek styles like Norfolk, safari, wrap, cardigan, belted, double breasted, hacking, mandarin, cowboy (especially when of fringed suede), jean (not blue), fur parka or vest, Spanish shawl, quilted bolero, cardigan sweater. **Shirts:** tailored, sexy, peasant and western, string sweater, tee, one-shouldered, V-neck, side-closing, unbuttoned. **Dresses:** shirt, peasant, tee, wrap, tunic, choengsam, caftan, kimono, toga, djellaba, one-shouldered, sweater knit. **Also:** jumpsuits, leopard-print lingerie, revealing robes. **Jeans:** Western, modified, cigarette (earth-toned, not blue denim). Look for satin jeans. **Pants:** slacks, drawstring, warm-up, jodhpurs, wrap, harem, skinny, tennis shorts in rough texture and/or earthy color, gym shorts, high leg/low neck maillots, also bandeau and string bikinis. **Skirts:** wrap, straight, full-circle, multi-tiered, sarong, slit.

— ACCESSORIES —

No other harmony has T-3's breadth of choice in accessories, especially jewelry. Lucky, lucky 3s! Your choices include:

Headgear: sportscar cap, watch cap, beret, snapbrim, coolie dish, tricorne, Panama, fedora, Russian sheepskin, southwester, cowboy, fur, Cossack, Chinese headdress, turban (especially lamé or brocade), rough straw, feathered, also trimmed with feathers or one long pheasant feather. In addition, Spanish combs, mantilla, chopsticks in hair. **Scarves and Ties:** knit, rough-textured choices in solid or paisley, diagonal stripe, patterns that lend movement without cuteness. **Watches:** square, rectangular, octagon, hexagon, with Roman numerals or dig-

ital, an alligator, pigskin or ostrich band. **Belts:** reptile with square or rectangular buckle would be a classic, but also rough leather, tooled, braided leather/ hemp-/straw, thong, exotic buckles, wrap and obi styles. **Bags and Wallets:** reptile, ostrich, pigskin-look, braided/woven/diagonal details, rough-surfaced leather, tooled leather, canvas, homespun, straw, brocade and tortoiseshell. Designed with angles (not curves), worn bandolier style, on shoulder, arm, in hand or pocket. **Shoes:** diagonal lines, detailing or trim in calf, suede, reptile, wood. Best shades are cordovan, brown, rust, camel and metallics. Look for boots with textural interest, ankle to thigh lengths, brogue, oxford, wingtip, tie, huarache, moccasin, loafer, sandal, slide. Seek moccasin toe, stacked heel, X banded vamp, kiltie flap, square or rectangular buckle, heavy hardware and crepe/rope/or bamboo-covered soles. Shoes should be earthy or sexy in appearance, not delicate. Textured hose for daytime is great—so are argyles. **Jewelry:** all the metals—copper, nickel, brass, bronze, gold, silver, platinum—worked in unusual, asymmetric designs. Choose antique, hammered, encrusted effects. Lion's head, temple dragon or serpent designs, heavy squash-blossom necklace, celtic cross, carved ivory, scrimshaw, rough beads, baroque pearls, jade, topaz, tiger's eye, tortoise, malachite, garnet, rough coral, rock, wood, bone, seed, shell, jute, straw, cork, leather, horsehair, bamboo, macramé, jungle or animal themes, plus hammered rectangular earrings or gypsy hoops, arm bracelets, wire spiral bracelets, multiple chains. Mix different metals in same costume.

As Type Four needs to remove jewelry before leaving home, Type Three needs to add. You can handle more texture and detail than any other harmony . . . look plain without it.

One more group and you'll have the entire picture. Type Four steps front-center in the next chapter.

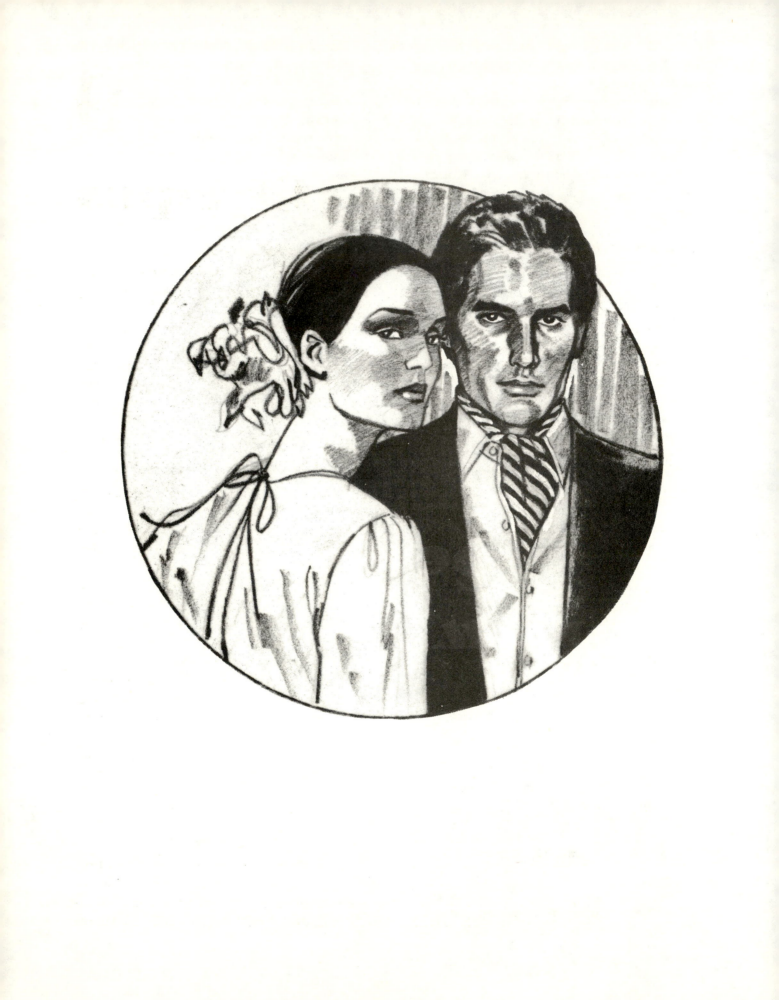

9

Olympus

Grecian columns of pristine marble bridge earth and heaven in formal grace. Type Four gods and goddesses glide regally through vaulted halls, raven locks hosting diadems, flowing draperies reflecting light. Features are beautifully sculpted, brows—noble, eyes—profound.

Olympians exude the mystery and magnetism associated with uniqueness and beauty. Deep emotions hide within these cool intellectuals, neither hot-blooded outburts nor impetuous gestures disturb their serenity.

Leaving the temple of the gods for the twentieth century is but a short step for Type Fours. They retain a clarity of mind which sets them apart as completely as does their beauty.

Visual contrast is the one item common to all T-4s, but it comes in different forms. Most obvious form is value contrast: dark hair and eyes/light skin or dark hair, skin and eyes/light teeth and whites-of-the-eye. Other forms of contrast include: cool eyes/warm skin, warm eyes/cool skin or the intensity contrast of electric eyes/still face. Sound like a lot of variety? It is, even though Type Fours are somewhat rare. Sorry, no natural towheads or redheads here.

Let's compare and contrast Type Four. As with the other harmonies, T-4s are arranged from largest to smallest in size and strongest to least strong in impact.

Electra and Conrad are tall and slender with aristocratic noses and some angularity of face. Formal, sophisticated, aloof—they don't need anyone's approval. High fashion is their forte as are extremes in line, contrast, silhouette and accessory. Nothing soft or indecisive here.

Less dramatic and having a different beauty, Serena and Blake, apparent graduates of a proper finishing school, boast smoother skin, lighter eyes (perhaps blue), and oval faces. Elegant and well-bred, they choose beautiful fabrics in well-designed styles . . . the understated classic which appears expensive and can be worn for years.

Diane and Michael are wider and squarer, less delicate and refined, more approachable and natural. Most comfortable in elegantly casual styles, they leave the drawingroom sleekness and high-fashioned clothing to their taller cousins.

Jocelyn and Wayne are soft, more rounded in form, with long-lashed eyes, even features and graceful movements. Faces, figures and coloring are highly decorative so this type, especially, must keep clothing simple.

Smallest of the T-4s are Laura and Drew. Like ballet dancers, they're small-boned, trim and compact. As potential for drama lowers, costumes simplify and contrast lessens.

The T-4s verging on other harmonies may occasionally borrow details to add to a total look but *never* in violation of T-4's sophistication.

— COLORS —

Type Four colors are cool, still and brilliant . . . fire locked inside a block of ice or flashes from sunlight through a crystal. Winter's cold and sparkle is enhanced by silvery tones plus whites, blacks and clear grays. High intensity forms of red, purple, blue, turquoise, green and yellow give the quality of illuminated stained-glass or most beautiful jewels. Page 41 lists T-4 colors.

T-4s use contrast to reinforce their look: black/white, bright blue/white, chrome yellow/black, emerald green/hot pink.

T-4s use unequal amounts of two colors.

T-4s avoid blended, earthy and muddy colors.

— FABRICS —

These fabrics lend the "born with a silver spoon" look that T-4s seek:

suede, Ultrasuede, fine wool flannel, menswear, wool crepe, wool challis and jersey, velvet, velveteen, velour, brushed denim, no-wale or finewale corduroy, crisp knits, linen, cotton, silk jacquard, finest silk or silver brocade, silver lamé, satin, delusterized satin, taffeta, crepe de chine, crepe, Nyesta, Qiana, silk, handkerchief linen, voile, mousseline, charmeuse, shadow-striped chiffon, delicate crystal beading, lavishly used sequins and "glitter" like powdered snow.

— LEATHERS AND FURS —

City sophisticates, Type Fours need striking and expensive-looking furs to frame smooth skin, regular features and cool elegance. Best choices include:

ermine, lustrous dark or white mink, black or silver fox, gray chinchilla, dark Russian sable, Russian Broadtail, Swakara or Karakul lamb, opossum and fisher.

Garments should be either high-fashion styling or elegantly classic. Fur capes, coats, jackets, linings, boas, collars, hats, bags all should be considered.

Leathers include smooth, finely-textured, suede, calf, patent and kidskin.

Avoid patterned furs, rough skins, young styles or anything appearing inexpensive.

— FABRIC DESIGNS —

Since *line* is your most important element, you would usually choose smooth sol-

ids. But there are becoming prints. Look for relaxed, calm, still, restful effects such as:

geometrics: shadowstripe, pinstripe, linestripe, unevenly-spaced stripes, houndstooth, tattersall, line plaids and black and white windowpane checks (avoid the look of checkered tablecloths).

Abstracts: choose tasteful designs like marble, weeping willows, mountains and valleys, and good abstracts.

Avoid the ordinary, cute, rough and pretty.

Avoid unbecoming colors, wrong scale (too large or small for you), and poor design.

— GARMENT DETAILING —

As with Type Two, Type Four seeks oval lines but uses them with discretion, less lavishly. Look for distinctive lines having curved lapels and seaming, oval necklines and detailing, but KEEP DETAIL TO A MINIMUM. You want the fewest, most invisible closures, pockets, belts and buttons.

Necklines: simplicity of the ascot . . . best of all possible styles . . . plus slim mandarin, slash, oval, draped, cowl, jewelry, turtle or strapless. **Collars:** oval, shawl, notched, shirt, ascot-tied, bertha. **Sleeves:** Long, set-in, cuffed, occasionally an extreme design like a batwing. **Also:** empire waist-lines, floating panels, flowing and slim lines, some narrow piping, tasteful trapunto.

Avoid ruffles, bows, embroidery, monograms and fringe.

Avoid skimpily-cut garments, inexpensive designs and poor workmanship.

— TYPES OF CLOTHING —

A wardrobe of costumes is your goal . . . not costumes in the sense of make-believe but in the sense of being totally coordinated. Separates are fine if pulled-together with vest, jacket, or accessories to give an elongated line and balanced silhouette. You can live with fewer clothes than any other harmony, but *yours have to look expensive.*

What should you choose?

Capes: street and floor lengths that coordinate with your outfit, have ample cut and drama. **Coats:** trim topcoat, wrap, trench, princess, spencer, duster, chesterfield, kimono-wrap, oversized poncho. Consider a silvery-satin trench or a fabulous cut-velvet wrap coat for evening. **Jackets:** blazer, hacking, spencer, bolero, tuxedo. **Suits:** European cut, American cut, tuxedo, tails, blazer. Choose vertical seaming and slash, not patch, pockets. **Shirts:** classic, turtleneck, cowl, tucked, ascot-tied, elongated tunic. **Dresses:** Grecian drape, empire, princess, cowled sweater, two and three piece knits, fitted, choengsam, strapless. **Also:** shawl-collared, satin-piped, long wrap robe; silken nightgown or pjs; slender caftan; maillot; white terry, shawl-collared, short beach wrap. **Jean:** straight-legged velvet, velveteen, satin, brushed denim. **Pants:** slacks, high-waist, straight leg, disco. **Skirts:** straight, wrapped, paneled, slightly flared, slightly gathered. Wear formal attire whenever possible.

— ACCESSORIES —

As previously mentioned, Types Two and Four need luxurious accessories to complete their "costumes." Type Fours choose from the following:

Headgear: sportscar cap, watchman's cap, homburg, beret, turban, dome, helmet, stiff cartwheel, wide-brimmed straw, fur hood. Trimmings should be self-color or eliminated. Jewelry *can* be worn in her hair and the tiara is hers alone!

Scarves and Ties: lightweight, smooth-surfaced, semi-crisp materials in your solid colors or prints. Look for ascots but also silk or cashmere mufflers, long scarves of self-fabric to wrap around hair or neck, ties in silk or silk-look that contrast with shirts. Ties may be solid, tone-on-tone, pin-striped, regimental stripes, club or ivy-league styles. **Watches:** oval, of polished silver or platinum—that expensive look! Fine leather strap. **Belts:** black calf as first choice with a self buckle. Cummerbunds are great. And for her, either an unobtrusive belt or the smashing waist ornament that "makes" her costume. **Bags and Wallets:** smooth black calf is perfect for secretary wallet or attache case for either sex, if unadorned. Outside of business, look for ovalized lines in simple clutch, envelope or shoulder bags. Materials may be calf, suede, satin, velvet, ottoman, beads or silver. **Shoes:** simple styles having elegance and grace. Fine calf slipons, cap toes and dress boots or slippers work for him. A graceful pump or delicate sandal is appropriate for her. Choose from calf, kid, patent or suede.

Avoid heavy, flashy or poorly-made footwear.

Jewelry: limited to *only ONE important piece for any outfit.* Look for strong, clean shapes. Wear a finely-crafted, highly-polished silver arm-bracelet with that perfect dress. Or let your decoration be a magnificent belt, squash-blossom necklace, breathtaking ring, tiara, *or* an antique from a queen's treasury. Earrings include half-moons, buttons or drops which do not swing or make a sound. Look for sculptured, smooth, body jewelry, shiny oval pendants, pins and rings, matched strands of pearls/jet beads/crystal beads, silver chains and settings of onyx, sapphine, star sapphire, ruby, emerald or diamond. The solitaire—emerald, marquis or brilliant cut—should be as large a "rock" as you can manage. Mix diamonds with rubies, emeralds or sapphires. Yours are the icy jewels. Rejoice!

Flowers rarely make a sophisticated statement. Use only if bold or unusual.

Avoid the cute, small, country and inexpensive. Gloves: wear, whenever they're in style, for gloves finish your costume. Walking umbrellas and walkingsticks also add panache.

You've worked your way through the selections belonging to your harmony, but you can't LOOK LIKE YOURSELF AND LOVE IT! without even more input. Luckily, it follows!

How Do You
Select It?

## 10

Wardrobes: Wonderful or Woeful?

Wonderful wardrobes aren't created by unlimited funds and massive quantities of clothes, much as you might like to believe it. There's a far more important element. Key to a wonderful wardrobe—with a flattering costume for every occasion—is DISCIPLINE. There is no substitute. Neither Fort Knox's gold nor Cher's looks can compensate for a lack of discipline.

How do you gain discipline? You *have it already* when your goals become more important than the current temptation . . . be it a chocolate doughnut, a sale-priced snakeskin belt, *another* late night or ignoring your exercise program.

The first step to your super wardrobe:

— A DISCIPLINED CLOSET —

With at least two uninterrupted hours, first, remove *everything* from your closet. Next, cover bed and chair with hanging items . . . the floor with everything else.

Now, dust and vacuum, scrub woodwork and replace shelf paper. Make your closet shine. You can also paint or paper the walls, but this takes prior planning, supplies and additional time.

With good light, inspect each item of apparel and sort them into seven groups.

1. Those with worn areas.
   Those which don't fit.
   Those which are out-of-style
   Those unworn during the past year.
2. Wearable items needing a stitch, a button, new heels.
3. Wearable items needing laundering.
4. Wearable items needing dry cleaning.
5. Wearable items needing pressing.
6. Wearable items needing polishing: shoes, boots, attaches, bags.
7. Wearable items that are currently wearable.

Return group 7 to your closet. Attend to groups 2-6 but forbid them space beside your wearables. NO PARKING ALLOWED until clothes which need attention receive it.

If you can't sew, barter with someone for that service. You can offer a meal, car wash, or babysitting. Or, take your to-be-remodeled/mended items to your local cleaners. Most have alteration services.

Now to group 1—

Items that are worn out have earned retirement. Save handsome buttons for a later use. Save soft and absorbent garments for dustcloths and car rags. Copy or have copied any style you can't live without, but not before you've completed this book and reevaluated. You could change your mind in the interim.

Items which don't fit or are out-of-style should be altered, given away or stored. Banish shoe mistakes—hurting shoes show on your face. Gifts to charitable organizations are tax deductible, so donate your clothing, get a receipt for its value, and state that amount as a deduction at tax time. Store clothing in far-removed places like Aunt Susie's attic. Never let unnecessary boxes invade your living space.

Otherwise wearable items unworn during the past year can be studied. Why haven't you worn it? Unflattering color? Unbecoming lines? Too identifiable? Not elegant? No accessories to wear with it? After you understand your aversion, can its style be altered, will it work with a vest, a tunic, new accessories? If it won't ultimately delight you, not just be tolerated, dump it, pronto.

You might enjoy a quote by Ida Bailey Allen, "The difference between most of us and the 'ten best dressed women' is that we can not afford to discard mistakes, while they can not afford to wear them." But if you love yourself, you, also, can't afford to wear mistakes nor to make them on your new selections.

Now, look at your neat, semi-bare closet. Are clothes droopng from wire hangers? Splurge on attractive wood or plastic hangers that lend better support. Coats and jackets need shaped hangers. Pants, shirts and shorts hang best on clampstyle hangers. All garments must be straight on the hanger with buttons and zippers fastened. "Like" items—all jackets—hang together, not with their vests and pants. This encourages you to dream up combinations you'd never think of if garments hang as sets.

Furs are cleaned, glazed and stored in the summer, and each requires its own padded, shaped hanger and *cloth* covering for the cool weather. Never cover with plastic!

How about accessories? Look through your belts, scarves, ties and jewelry. Sort and weed as you did with your clothes. Keep the good-but-not-fashionable items, and take them out of storage when they return to vogue.

Lay wearable sweaters and knit items on shelves or in drawers or boxes. Place wearable jewelry pieces into individual niches to prevent scratches. Hang easily-tangled chains from a tie bar. Have any loved and often worn costume jewelry copied in precious metal. You'll enjoy it all your life.

Hang your four most-often-worn belts on a coat hook. The rest, grouped by color, go into plastic shoe boxes.

Install another closet shelf above your existing one, the height of your shoes plus one-inch between. This upper shelf holds storage items and allows your shoes their own space, off the floor, where you can easily see them. Slip odor-proof liners into any shoes that could benefit.

An alternate plan, or one for a second closet, includes adding a rod just the height of your shirts from the floor. Then raise the existing rod enough to allow for double-decker space. Clothes need air and freedom from bunching.

Arrange space outside your closet for clothing which needs attention. *Never return anything to your closet that isn't in top shape.* Hang wrinkled garments in your bathroom while you shower. This eliminates some pressing. By keeping non-perfect items out of your closet, you can always count on those items within.

To complete your closet inventory, list your *wearables* on the following charts. Pencil a word or two (red corduroy) in the appropriate space (jacket).

You'll return to this chart many times in the future to make additions or substitutions, to plan your wardrobe in detail and to check on the specifics of your next purchase. You might find it helpful to duplicate or copy the chart. Having it on a sheet of paper would increase its convenience and portability, allowing you to tuck it in purse or pocket, erase, jot notes in the margin, whatever.

Ideal selections for average wardrobes follow in the next chapter. Don't miss them.

PERSONAL WARDROBE CHART

ITEM	HAVE	NEED
COATS JACKETS WRAPS		
SUITS		
BLOUSES SHIRTS SWEATERS —SEPARATES— SLACKS SKIRTS SHORTS		

ITEM	HAVE	NEED
DRESSES DRESS-UP CLOTHES		
ACTIVE SPORT		
SCARVES JEWELRY		
BELTS BAGS WALLETS		
SHOES		
SOCKS		
UNDER CLOTHES		
AT-HOME SLEEPWEAR		

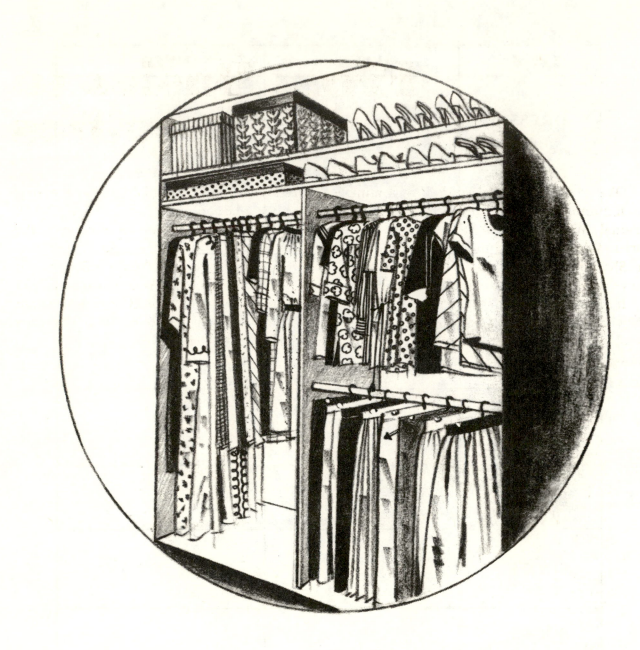

11
From Basics to Specifics

Okay, you've stripped yourself to a minimum number of clothes and accessories Your *Personal Wardrobe Chart* has mighty few entries. When's the shopping trip? Sorry, not yet. Shopping is the last step in a series and you've only completed the first few steps.

It's time to look at *Ideal Minimal Wardrobes*. These are designed for optimum coverage of unforeseen activities with a minimum number of pieces. Sound good? It is. It's the

perfect backbone on which to hang a new wardrobe plan.

You'll detect a resemblance between the *Ideal Minimal Wardrobe* and "basic" or "travel" wardrobes. They're all alike, give or take a few items, and worth using. If you begin with a compact wardrobe, you'll obtain more mileage from each garment and be ready for a major trip, instantly.

HER MINIMAL WARDROBE

1 coat (zip-lining ideal)
1 dark suit (dress up or down)
1 pantsuit or slacks or jeans
1 dress-up dress
1 dress (dress up or down)
1 knit or jersey dress
1 long skirt
3 blouses
1 sweater or sweater set
3 bras
3 slips
6 pair pantyhose
1 pair walking shoes
1 pair dress pumps or sandals
1 carryall handbag
1 dress envelope bag
2 nightgowns or pajamas
1 lightweight robe, long, opaque
1 pair lightweight slippers
2 36" square scarves (bright)
1 swimsuit
1 pair dark glasses
1 shower cap
1 umbrella
accessories: belts, beads, jewelry, hats.

HIS MINIMAL WARDROBE

1 topcoat
1 dark suit
1 sport jacket
2 pair slacks
1 pair jeans or casual pants
3 dress shirts
1 sport shirt
1 sweater
4 ties
1 belt
4 sets underwear
6 handkerchiefs
6 pair of sox
2 pair of shoes
2 pair of pajamas
1 lightweight robe
1 pair lightweight slippers
1 pair swimtrunks
1 umbrella
1 hat (optional)
(Men are lucky!)

The preceding charts are only examples. Don't follow them religiously. The entire Four Harmony system is designed to assist you toward uniqueness, not confine you to a "rubber stamp" image.

If you shun sunning, swimming, lakes and seashores, you needn't invest in swimwear. If you live in jeans and interesting tops, you'll scratch the "establishment" items. Your list should fit YOU.

Remember the list is an excellent one for a major vacation unless you're biking through Scandinavia. Then, of course, you'd trim your list to not much more than the clothes on your back.

Lists can sound very barren. How does your suggested wardrobe list relate to the Four Harmonies? Each Type would obviously adapt it differently. Look at these possible interpretations.

Feel free to switch color families and styles in order to make the most of YOUR looks . . . but don't forget to choose garments that mix-and-match in the greatest number of combinations with the fewest accessories. This is imperative until you have an extensive wardrobe, all of which is perfect.

Neutrals are heavily used in the Wardrobe Examples because they're less remembered when you must wear them constantly. Also, they combine well with color or other neutrals and don't project a mood. Moods are covered in the *next* chapter.

Four Wardrobe Examples for HER

TYPE	ONE	TWO	THREE	FOUR
coat	butterscotch poplin pile-zipline trench	dove grey moire taffeta fur-zipline wrap	camel twill tweed-zipline trench	jet black gabardine fur-zipline wrap
suit	navy gabardine blazer	burgundy ultrasuede dressmaker	rust tweed dbl breasted	banker's grey worsted slimline
pants	blue denim jeans	gray flannel slacks	rust corduroy jeans	black velvet straight pants
after 5	turquoise silk full skirted creamy pearls	rose crepe draped pink pearls	bronze metallic-knit V-neck sheath exotic bib	black velvet empire sheath diamond clip
dress	lavender linen jacket dress	wedgewood challis shirtmaker	avocado raw silk wrap	white linen coatdress
tops	white dots on red tie silk bowed	pink chiffon scarfed	gold paisley knit wrap	white satin ascot
	lime cotton tee	gray charmeuse tunic	burnt orange raw silk shirt	chrome yellow silk shirt
	red pointelle sweater set	aqua cashmere cowl sweater	nubby brown V neck pullover	black turtleneck sweater
shoes	butterscotch calf mid-heel pump hi-heel sandal	taupe calf mh pump hh sandal	camel alligator pump copper/bronze crossstrap sandal	black calf mh pump hh silk sandal
hose	skintone	taupe	skintone	taupe
bras slips	young style skintone	lacy skintone	leopard see-thru	black white

70

Four Wardrobe Examples for HIM

TYPE	ONE	TWO	THREE	FOUR
top coat	beige twill trench	taupe cashmere wrap coat	chestnut rough wool Balmaccan	dark gray melton Chesterfield
suit	navy smooth blend blazer cut	dk. blue gray silk European cut	earthy herringbone British cut	charcoal pinstripe European cut
sport coat	beige flannel blazer	burgundy velvet belted-back	gold tweed Norfolk	black mohair blazer
slacks	grey flannel	maroon flannel	brown twill	light gray flannel
slacks	blue jeans	taupe flannel	rust corduroy	black & white houndstooth
dress shirts	pale blue pale gray cream	cream taupe silk blue-gray	gold homespun tattersall slub silk	white white on white pale blue
casual	western	ascot	thong-laced	silk turtle
ties	navy/white dots navy-red rep maroon club maroon solid	maroon/taupe ivy league maroon t/on/t taupe silk soft blue silk	paisley homespun textured plaid	blue silk club maroon silk knit gray solid white ascot scarf
shoe	black slip on	black cherry dress boot	brown brogue	black sleek captoe
socks	black mid-calf	maroon heather mid-calf	brown argyles	black mid-calf
sweater	gray wool crewneck	maroon silk turtle	rust tweed V-neck	black wool turtle

For now, think about your activities. What do you do? How do you spend your time? The following chart will inventory your time, assisting you to plan appropriate clothing for each activity and teaching where to place wardrobe emphasis.

To avoid confusion, two terms must be defined. "Dressing Down" doesn't indicate "grubbies," it means clothing appropriate for daytime and streetwear. "Dressing Up" refers to clothing appropriate for after-five dress or special daytime occasion wear.

Pencil your answers into the Personal Activities Analysis. On each line followed by an asterisk(*), indicate the appropriate number of times you engaged in that particular activity during the past year.

PERSONAL ACTIVITIES ANALYSIS

My occupation is _____
   (executive, brick layer, teacher, dentist, homemaker)
My ideal work uniform is_____ *
My ideal leisure clothes are _____ *
My sports include_____ *
My lounging clothes are _____ *
My home entertaining is formal_____ *   casual_____ *
                       informal_____ *   patio_____ *
                       sport oriented_____ *

My "Dress Down" activities include:
   meetings & lectures_____ * casual luncheons_____ *
   shopping (not for groceries)_____ * movies_____ *
   spectator sport_____ *   casual dinners_____ *
My "Dress Up" activities include:
   cocktail parties_____ * dinner dancing_____ * disco_____ *
   restaurant/hotel dining_____ * theatre/opera_____ *
   formal or holiday dinner parties in private homes _____ *
     gala occasions (formal balls, first nights) _____ *
My travel is by: plane_____ * train_____ * car_____ *
   ship_____ *
My vacations are spent: on a cruise_____ * touring_____ *
   at a resort_____ * pursuing a sport_____ *
   camping_____ * seeing foreign country_____ *

Note those areas of heavy activity. If you spend every day on the tennis court you'll need more tennis gear, from shoes through warmups. Now turn back to your Personal Wardrobe Chart on pages 66-67 and:

1. Star those *areas* of heaviest use.
2. Pencil-in the wardrobe you would need to be well-dressed for each occasion. Keep this list as short as possible. *The smaller your wardrobe the easier it is to maintain.* This is one time that "less is more."
3. Check your present clothing and accessories against your Becoming Color Collection from Chapter 6. Place a *plus* (+) by items of a becoming color. Place a *minus* (-) beside items of an unbecoming color.
4. Inventory your present wardrobe list again and add a plus (+) for each item which fits as a part of your Minimal Wardrobe.

5. Check your "Need" write-ins to see that they coordinate with the *plus* items you own. Minus garments and accessories will ultimately be replaced with something better.

The majority of readers have fewer than five perfect items left when they finally understand what they could be doing for themselves. If you have more than five, congratulations! If you have fewer, you're in for exciting change.

In Chapter Twelve you'll learn how to dress for special occasions. For instance . . .

12

Help, What Should I Wear???

What shall I wear??? is a universal question that appears with invitations, job interviews, all non-routine activities. And answers to that question needn't come from flipping a coin.

Begin with a primary rule: *Clothing choice should take into consideration the occasion, formality and setting, activities involved, time of day and year, climate, weather, and locality (including regional, national, and religious differences).*

Wow, with a rule like that it would seem you'd need a mammoth wardrobe, but not so! It merely means that high heels on a hike, wool "turtle" on a hot beach, or too-tight pants at a sit-on-the-floor party would be "out." Also "out" would be shorts in a country where native women wear dresses, strapless tops at church and shirtless torsos on the tennis court. In other words, USE COMMON SENSE.

When you're unable to ascertain the game plan beforehand, dress conservatively. You'll be more comfortable underdressed than overdressed. Pocketing your tie and opening your collar can lower the formality as switching to dressier shoes and jewelry can raise it—if that switch is possible.

— FOR JOB INTERVIEWS —

Check the field. See how others already working in that type of job dress. Now choose a conservative copy for yourself. Experts often list just what to wear for interviews, but if you dress expensively and the job pays a pittance, you'll not usually get on the payroll. There's one exception—if you're a receptionist.

Be scrupulous with your grooming whether your attire is strictly business or casual. Clothes must be pressed and spotless, nails neat and clean, hair attractive, makeup natural. In the get-a-job game NEATNESS COUNTS.

— FOR BUSINESS —

An Ideal Minimal Wardrobe has the beginning elements of a business wardrobe, but it's far from adequate if you work five days a week as a professional. More business clothes are needed and should be added to your collection as rapidly as possible.

Suits are usually first choice, but you can choose sportcoats and slacks, skirts and vests, or dresses if they are appropriate at your office. Check to see the quality and kind of clothing your immediate supervisor is wearing. Dress similarly if he/she is advancing in the company. If you want promotions, dress like the sharp people above you, not like those in your own or lower positions.

John T. Molloy, in his "Dress for Success" books, offers logical reasons for wearing a *uniform of success*, and I agree—up to a point. Men have worn suits and ties for ages—the price of promotion. That women should feel exempt from this form of dues-paying isn't logical.

Yet, individuals need alternatives. A prescribed "image" isn't the complete answer. Types One or Two won't reach the top of the company by wearing the uniforms of T-3s and T-4s. They'd look awful dressed in them.

Never step outside the clothes of your type for business or any other occasion. You can be a first rate _____ (supply your own harmony), but only a second or third rate any-other-type.

Always "mark" an outfit with the sign of your harmony. You may be wearing a neutral suit which could be worn by a variety of types. If so, make it your own with a tie, a scarf, a touch of brightness, a piece of jewelry—something which relates to your harmony and, thus, to you.

Choose the best quality you can afford. Business clothes are major investments that can last for years.

— FOR THE PODIUM —

When you are the speaker, trim your outfit to eliminate all distractions. This is *not* the time for busy prints, voluminous fabrics or noisy jewelry. Clothes will upstage you if you let them. It's the time for classic lines, becoming colors and quality.

If your audience is huge, see a stage makeup person. Special makeup will project your features beyond the tenth row.

— FOR TELEVISION APPEARANCES —

When you appear on television, dress as for the podium, with these exceptions. TV cameras don't register as wide a value (dark-/light) range as the eye; so avoid white, black, and combinations of the two. Bright colors containing yellow also flare, so avoid brightest lemon, lime and orange. Prints and dots disconcert the viewer—plain colors are preferable.

Mid-range neutrals, blue and colors containing blue are perfect for television. The light-to-medium blue shirt or blouse is classic.

Beware of revealing slits, distracting necklines and reflective or noisy jewelry.

You'll generally be "miked" with a tie-clasp style microphone. It mustn't be tucked under rustling taffeta nor bumped by jewelry. The soundman goes crazy when you add unnecessary noise.

You'll be responsible for your own makeup unless you appear on a national program. Use subtle contouring and a matte finish with carefully applied daytime makeup. Avoid white or shiny gleamers.

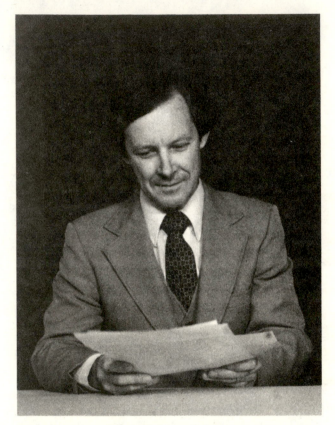

T-2 dressed for television

— FOR DRESS-UP —

Dress-up times call for richer fabrics, dressier designs and more luxurious jewelry. Best color choices are your "Elegant" ones. Choose neutrals only if you're willing to be invisible. (You'll be learning the language of color in the next chapter.)

White Tie on an invitation means the man should wear "tails," the woman her most magnificent creation. Large Balls are the most festive affair you'll ever attend . . . and they're coming back . . . so wear a spectacular gown.

Black Tie indicates he will wear a tuxedo, she a lovely evening gown.

Informal prescribes dark suit for him and short, dressy suit or dress for her.

If your wardrobe doesn't contain tails and tuxedo, they can be rented for special occasions. And women, short of magnificent creations, can combine a bare evening top with long skirt, bright cummerbund (if you have the proper waist, and stole. Be creative with flowers instead of jewels. You can look and feel gorgeous.

Morning weddings are the time for suits or simple dresses. Outdoor weddings are attended by men in light-toned suits, women in delicate dresses. Formal evening weddings call for dark suits for him, semi-covered long dresses for her. But check for regional differences.

— FOR FUNERALS —

Black is no longer required for funerals, fortunately. Men may wear a dark suit, light shirt, and dark tie, shoes and socks. Women should choose conservative, neutral clothing with a minimum of jewelry.

— FOR DRESS-DOWN —

Separates have become our "dress-down" uniforms and are joys to buy as well as own. The individual with widely varying measurements can find pants in one size and a jacket in another. It's far less expensive and much more satisfactory than hiring a tailor to do massive alterations. Separates in one's wardrobe greatly expand it. One jacket, two pair of pants and three tops doesn't equal six pieces . . . it can equal fourteen outfits . . . figuring all possible combinations of those garments. Watch that all your separates coordinate with each other, or you'll be left with just a few pieces rather than numerous outfits.

— FOR HOME AT-WORK —

Wielding hammer or skillet, lawnmower or vacuum, your clothing should be comfortable, practical and *bought for the purpose*. Relegating wornout finery to after-work hours is foolish. Clothing not made for the strain is rarely comfortable and will provide embarrassing should someone drop-in. Toss them, instead—the clothing, not the guest!

— FOR HOME AT-REST —

Besides having functional clothes for on the job and for household tasks, you'll undoubtedly need two kinds of relaxing clothes—the ultra comfortable and the "special."

The first could be a voluminous eye-color robe that cuddles you, a bright warmup suit or stretch-terry jumpsuit. When you don your comfortable garb, you should feel safe and cozy.

The second is for fantasy times when you'd like to project sexy, wealthy, elegant, or gorgeous. You could wear it alone, for your own pleasure, or when a friend drops by. Your "special" outfit may be caftan, satin lounging pajamas, a satin-bound robe, pegnoir and gown, whatever makes you feel valued and desirable.

Next area, a vital one, is the language of color. You mustn't miss it.

13 The Language of Color

How can color talk? When you sought your Becoming Colors you learned one color will sabotage you, the next flatter, the third just lie there. That's talking, of a sort, but it's not color's language.

Color talks by both establishing a mood and by projecting various facets of your personality. Your bright Becoming Colors are the vocal ones even though their message is given silently. What do they say?

Each color family sends a different message or mood to observers when you wear *its* color. By choosing a bright color you are, in fact, choosing a mood to project *and controlling how others see you.* Go through your color families and learn their various moods.

— EYE COLORS —

Your eye color projects a quiet, comfortable, approachable mood. It won't spotlight you or make you feel elegant, but it will be easy to wear—being especially kind when you feel swollen-faced from a cold. When you wear your eye color, others draw close, confide, expect your acceptance. It's a personal color that is nearer to being neutral than any of the other brights.

Use eye colors for "uniform" clothes such as riding pants, raincoat, go-everywhere pantsuit, work clothes and casuals.

— REDS —

Red is the color of life, fire, romance. It includes all the pinks through the oranges *that you can wear*. And don't think that this family of Becoming Colors belongs only to females. Color doesn't respect gender. There are no age or sex limitations. Everyone can and should wear some form of red when it is desirable to express femininity or masculinity. Red is the sex-oriented color you choose when you want to be seen by the opposite sex—a tremendous ego-boost at a party—it's magnetic. But a note of caution: spouses aren't the only ones to be turned-on by him in his ruby tie or scarlet vest, her in her rose tunic or twirly dress.

Red on a lawyer can sway opposite-sex jurors; on a salesman, his/her prospects; on a lover, the beloved. Enough said.

— LIMELIGHT COLORS —

There are times when you need to steal the show: when you want to be nominated or elected, when you're the guest of honor or the speaker, when you would be "star" of the party. Whenever you want to look better than you've ever looked and aren't afraid to show it, wear your highest mood or your *Limelight* colors. This family of colors places your coloring in the spotlight, heightening and dramatizing your hair, eyes, skin and lips—drawing attention magnetically.

A word of warning: this type of attention is best when your grooming is immaculate, your costume perfect. Otherwise the attention might not be completely comfortable. But, again, you won't always be wearing your Limelight color from head-to-toe. They're superb choices in scarves, ties, shirts and jewelry—super brighteners for your neutrals.

What are your Limelight colors? Most people look their smashingest in the yellow-green/green/blue-green family of colors. These colors are across the color wheel from your skin color's position and complementary colors intensify each other.

But if you have unusual coloring, your Limelight colors may fall in the blue/blue-violet/violet family. You'll have to try both sets and see. When the cooler group does most for you, switch Limelight and Elegant colors and go on like everyone else.

— ELEGANT COLORS —

What if you *don't* want the spotlight? What if "second fiddle" is your role? At these ceremonial times: weddings, christenings, anniversary parties, receptions, a quieter image is more appropriate. Besides, to the bride, the baby, the anniversary couple, the honorees belongs stage center. You'll enjoy looking refined and attractive.

When your boss gives the talk at the luncheon or your spouse is the guest-of-honor, or you attend church or the opera, choose your Elegant colors and mood-dress for the occasion. You'll look both super and appropriate.

Elegant colors generally include the blue/blue-violet/violet tones that look great on you. They have a quiet, cool, restraining effect that's flattering, but more refined than dramatic.

Never consider wearing a color that's outside your Becoming Color list, no matter what its mood. When blue is mentioned as being ideal, you need to interpret that as one of your icy pale blues or brilliant sapphires if you're a T-4, one of your blue-purples like fall grapes or the blue-greens of oxidized copper if you're a T-3. T-2s picture their soft wedgwoods or blue-grays, T-1s their crayon blues or blue mists.

Everyone can wear some shade or tint of every color, but each person's choice is differ-ent. People in the same harmony will wear more similar blues than those in differing harmonies, but they'll rarely be identical.

— UPLIFTING COLORS —

When your mood or your appointment's mood is "black" or "down," wear one of your yellows. This may be gold/yellow/yellow-orange/yellow-green/lemon/marigold/orange, whichever shade or tint yours happen to be. Wearing warm yellow is like wearing sunshine. It will lift the spirits of all who see you. Rainy days, visiting the sick, the bereaved, working with children, blue Mondays—all improve with the addition of this happy, "up" color family.

— NEUTRALS —

Neutrals are all the dull, non-bright colors that become you, whether light, mid-range or dark. They are silent colors that project no mood.

Neutrals are less noticed than your bright colors; so they make excellent wardrobe extenders. You could wear a gray jacket every day for a week, and no one would notice if your shirts and scarves/ties/jewelry and pants/skirts were different. Neutrals figure heavily in a Minimal Wardrobe for this very reason.

Use small touches of different brights to alter the mood of your neutral costumes. The same suit can project all the moods by changes in accessories.

Avoid neutrals when you go to parties. Neutrals are impersonal and you want your personality displayed when you party.

Your darkest neutral (black?) with your lightest of that family (silver gray?) is the most formal and businesslike combination you can wear—absolutely perfect for borrowing money from the bank. You'll look all business, for your personality will be hidden.

Neutrals with more color—blue-gray, dark teal, pale cinnamon, maroon, deep plum—are less formal than the businesslike black. Light colors are less formal than dark.

If you'd be considered an authority, choose a dark, lapeled jacket to add weight to your statements.

— COLOR PREFERENCE —

Perhaps you've always loved green and hated red. Should you stick with the colors you love and exclude the others? Definitely not. Your liking for a color is unrelated to its becomingness. You usually like or dislike colors because of happy or unhappy experiences in the past.

Beloved Aunt Mary adored strawberry pink. The rooms of her home bloomed with berries; she wore the color at every opportunity, and plied you with strawberry shortcake whenever in season. Do you wonder the color warms and pleases you?

But if that pink were the color of a nasty medicine or the shirt of someone who scared you when you were younger, you'd react differently to it now.

Test colors on yourself, when your mood is *up*. Be objective. A color you've always worn and loved may not be becoming if you look at it critically. Conversely, a color you've always detested may be smashing on you.

— ADDITIONAL COLOR FACTS —

Avoid costumes which are half one color, half another. Keep amounts uneven. Use lots of one, a little of a second and a tiny dab of a third if you use three colors.

Avoid more than three colors in a costume.

An "accent" color is limited to TWO places—never a red belt, red tie and red hat at the same time.

Your warm and bright colors advance, lending a friendly, direct, personal aura. Use them for parties, play, beachwear and in small amounts with neutrals.

Your cool and dull colors recede, projecting refinement, reserve and conservativeness. Use for ceremonial and quiet occasions.

Strong contrast is magnetic, positive, attention getting. Some contrast is desirable in a costume, but unless you are a T-4, highest contrasts are best avoided. *You* must star, not your costume.

The larger the area the less intense its color should be. This is a safe rule. Break it only if you have a good reason plus a good figure.

The duller the color the more luxurious the fabric must be.

Monochromatic ensembles (varying shades of one color) need variety in texture or intensity, since they, by definition, have no variety of hue.

Remember, an almost-right color isn't as good as a "right" one on you. The former could sabotage, at worst, and at best it will remain an "outsider" in your family of clothes. Everything else will go together and the not-quite-right color will go with nothing else.

# # # # #

You may put your new color knowledge to work. Turn back to your Personal Wardrobe Chart on pages 66-67. Examine your lists of *Have* and *Need*. Are they the *best* colors for your purpose, considering color moods? Change the *Need* list again if necessary. It should reflect your best judgment of both items and colors that would be most becoming and practical for your purpose.

It's easy to erase one color and substitute another when you're working on paper but not so easy when the garment hangs in your closet. You're surely facing a very important question. "Do you make new purchases that combine with your present wardrobe but don't do the most for you, or do you choose new items that are perfect but stand alone?" The farther apart the two appear the more difficult the decision, but there can only be one answer.

Let the new items be perfect, even if it means disregarding the old wardrobe.

You can't *discard* the old wardrobe unless you have far more funds than most, but you can work around it. Let your first purchases be scarves or ties or shirts in your Becoming

Colors. By using "super" colors near your face you'll look far better and your old wardrobe can't last forever. As you replace wornout garments, you'll add great new ones and in a few years your personal wardrobe will delight and thrill you.

Shopping secrets come in the next chapter, so *please* don't buy anything major yet. The chapter on Disguise and Display also contains information you need to make wise purchases.

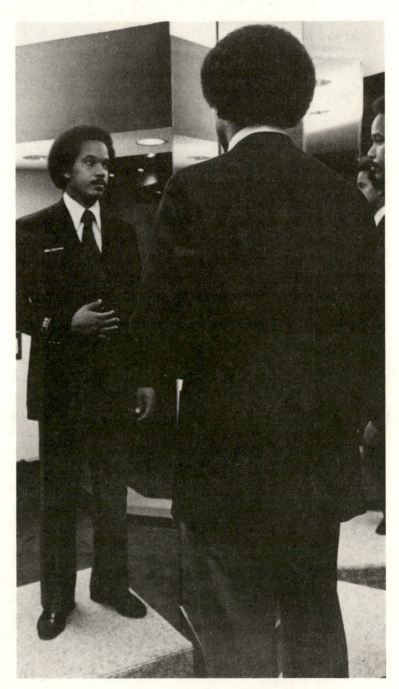

T-1 checking jacket for fit

14

Shopping Secrets

With jingling change in your jeans, you're off to replenish your wardrobe. But, to save time, money and energy, stock up on shopping secrets before you go.

Dress well for shopping. When you look sharp you'll have more energy, be equipped to determine becomingness and succeed with salespeople. "Tacky" won't do!

Have your hair stylist make necessary changes *before* you shop for a new season's clothes. Proportions are constantly shifting, and you can more easily balance your ensemble if your hair volume and line are established. Don't laugh. This is important.

Take-alongs. Shop only if you have your Becoming Colors in pocket or purse. You'll need money or charge cards, of course, but even more important, have a specific plan. Know what you need, possible colors, and approximate cost. You'll find this information, except for the cost, on your Personal Wardrobe Chart. Without data you're ripe for the impulse purchases which strip both clothes budgets and bodies.

Carry additional shoes if needed to accessorize the anticipated purchase, special socks if you're buying cowboy boots or tennis shoes, and the proper undergarments for new items. Shop in an outfit as similar to the one you're buying as possible—suit, shirt, tie, dress shoes when you're buying a suit. Be fitted in the clothes you'll be wearing under a topcoat, a vest. Never shop for dress clothes while treading in "Hush Puppies®."

Think ahead and, like the Scouts, "Be prepared."

Watch charge accounts. Nothing is more convenient, but if you pay finance charges, you're wasting your clothing dollar. Settle your old accounts, for interest rates on store charges are some of the highest known.

Shop when you are rested and have sufficient time. You'll be making important decisions and need your faculties well-honed. Avoid rush hours and pre/post Christmas crowds to gain the best service from clerks. Always treat your salesperson courteously.

Shop the best time for your harmony. Look for young, crisp, T-1 colors and styles in January when the spring clothing arrives. Summer clothes are most likely to be soft and romantic for T-2s. They're shown after Easter. Called fall fashions, textured and earthy clothes which best display T-3 become available in mid-summer. Chic and striking winter styles, appearing in November, are preferred choices for T-4s.

Buy all your brightly colored items and most of your neutrals during *your* season. Choose a variety of weights for year-round wear.

Shop before the season for greatest selection. When snow flies, the winter coat rack is nearly depleted. Shop for a warm coat in early August. Choose your swimwear in February.

Shop sales for lowest prices. Look for sales after Christmas, Easter, July Fourth, Labor Day, and on the last day of every month. But, an item is only a bargain if needed, in perfect condition, a proper fit, will remain in style for the next three years, will bridge seasons, can be worn/carried enough to make it inexpensive, reinforces your image, and is WANTED.

Shop when you need nothing. Finding a clothing store which stocks *your* kind of garments and accessories at *your* price is even better than locating a stupendous buy. Visit all the men's or women's clothing departments in each major department store. Check boutiques, exclusive salons, discount houses, catalogs, government surplus, and used clothing marts. Both bridal and loungewear sections hold potential eveningwear, and the teen departments for both sexes can net low-cost, classic finds.

Check current magazines to identify trends, see how items and colors are combined in a costume, and to determine the elements of "today's" look. Without proper imput, your purchases can look out-of-date before you've worn them.

When you locate the perfect store, ask the manager to recommend a salesperson. Let Mr/Ms Salesperson know your current and future needs. If you two are compatible, your new representative will be thinking of your requirements whenever new shipments arrive, putting-back items you might like, phoning when ordered items are delivered. You, in turn, can contact him/her when a special need arises and quickly ascertain your favorite store's ability to help.

Comparison shop for the look of quality. The more limited your clothing budget, the more necessary it is to shop expensive stores to see how well-designed, well-made garments look. Note the tailoring, the feel, the way it is lined, the overall impression. Try items on and see how they fit. Note which designs are flattering, which aren't. Measure significant details and copy them in garments you sew yourself. Have ready-mades altered to fit and look like the more expensive. By comparison shopping you learn to recognize top quality and can then interpret it in your price range.

Shop first for major purchases. Coats and suits fall into this category and should be chosen before you choose shirts and ties, blouses and accessories. But only buy coats and suits if they fit your lifestyle. Sunbelt areas make an extensive coat wardrobe unnecessary and the non-professional may need only one suit in his/her closet.

Choose interchangeables that will work several ways in YOUR wardrobe, can be dressed up or down, and will bridge at least three seasons.

Budget for your purchases. Check your Wardrobe Needs again; they're listed on pages 66-67. Now estimate the cost of each to-be-purchased item and pencil it in. Impulse purchases can easily waste 50 percent of your clothing funds. Don't let them!

Newspaper ads give prices, a quick breeze through stores will update your information, or a major chain catalog is an excellent, quick reference.

Allow most of your money for *major* purchases, for example: 1/5 of budget for coat, 1/5 of budget for suit, 1/5 of budget for 2 dresses, sport coat and slacks, or for an additional suit, 2/5 of budget for shoes, shirts, ties, belts, bags, hats and jewelry. Belts, bags, shoes and jewelry should *be* expensive. Shirts, blouses, scarves and ties should *look* expensive.

Spend most for clothes to be worn the most. A good rule is to divide purchase price by total number of wearings to determine cost-per-wearing of any item. In this manner a suit which costs $300 but is worn twice a week for five years costs only 60¢ per wearing plus cleaning fees. The party dress that cost only $25 and was worn twice cost $12.50 per wearing. Which was the better buy?

Love it or leave it. Neither closets nor budgets should be asked to house clothing which is so-so, that doesn't light up your eyes. Every day for years you'll delight in wearing a particular purchase, look and feel great in it, and be free to concentrate on something other than your appearance. Conversely, buy something for purely utilitarian reasons and you'll tolerate or eventually hate it. Joy will be diminished rather than increased.

Perhaps a beige, zip-lined trenchcoat is more practical, but a forest green greatcoat or ruby wool melton could steal your heart and warm it for years.

Invest in basics, not fads. The former never is out-of-style; the latter is dated in months. A fad is an unusual item that bursts into popularity and fades as soon as the majority possess it.

A classic suit or dress can stay in style for up to seven years; the novelty item can be an embarrassment within the year.

Buy at the beginning of a trend. Ties widen then narrow to widen again. Emphasis flits from hem to waist to shoulder to leg. But, fortunately, changes take time to sweep throughout the Western world and the average life of a major trend is seven years. Your security comes in knowing what's happening.

Plan on wearing new clothes a *minimum* of three years. The first two years be ahead of the masses; the last year everyone will have caught up, and you can begin researching fashion direction and upgrading once more. A word of caution: business clothes need to be conservative; so don't have the narrowest or widest anything. Go classic, classic, classic!

Don't sew with old fabric or patterns. Just as clothing ages, so do patterns and fabric. You want a *new* garment, not an unworn one which looks five years old.

Select one from a thousand. Each season a thousand separate ideas will be begging for adoption . . . placement of a slit, newest fashion color, "in" jewelry. Screen carefully and invest only in the absolutely perfect. Not perfect as a fashion idea but perfect for YOU. Everyone else may be wearing wide shoulders and pegged pants, but if this isn't the silhouette that becomes you, pass it over and adopt another look. Screen all possibilities. You'll find an adaptation that's flattering, and you'll have more than a fashion look, you'll have STYLE.

Check labels for fiber content, color fastness, estimated shrinkage, laundering and ironing requirements. All are important to a long love affair with your clothing. Cleaning fees can multiply a shirt's annual cost; and natural cotton, comfortable and fashionable though it be, can force more time at the ironing board or the laundry than you'll want to give.

Inspect each item for quality workmanship. Look for straight, even machine stitching; ample seam allowances and hems; reinforced points of strain such as armholes, waist, and button/buttonhole areas; plaids, stripes and large designs matched at seams; and zippers which lie flat and work easily.

Use a 3-way mirror to check fit. Sit, walk, bend, stretch in any garment you're considering. Discomfort will kill enjoyment.

Necklines and shoulders are the most important areas to check, the hardest to alter successfully and the areas most readily noticed since they're at eye-level.

Sleeves should be set without puckers, hang without wrinkles and allow full arm movement.

Darts take up material in hollow areas and release it at round ones. They should point toward but stop short of your body's fullest point. Bust darts too high? Too low? See if fabric has been clipped within the dart. If not, there is a possibility of alteration.

Expect alterations and add their cost to the price of each garment. The more figure irregularities you have, the more "fitting" you'll require.

Add quality to readymade clothes. Restitch seams which are poorly sewn or carry stress. Retack loosely-held buttons. Restitch buttonholes, if needed. Rehem if uneven or stitching shows. Tie stray threads and clip short. Remove string beltloops; they're designed for on-the-rack convenience, not for wearing. Remove tacky trimming—cheap buttons, belts, bows—replace with quality trimming which are appropriate to your harmony.

— WHAT TO AVOID —

The third costume in any category unless you spend most of your time in that activity.

Non-functioning details . . . non-buttoning buttons, non-pocket pockets, non-placket plackets, and raincoats that don't keep you dry.

Bold stripes. These too-often upstage the figure. Choose stripes as trimmings and the narrow, low contrast forms seen in men's better shirts.

Uncomfortable shoes. They'll show on your face.

White shoes and white handbags. Unless worn with slacks, white shoes make you look bottom-heavy. Choose skintone shoes and bags instead. They're less easily soiled and far more elegant.

Clear plastic raincoats and handbags.

— WEARING YOUR PURCHASES —

Dress rehearse before important functions. Try on your new outfit and view it critically from all angles. Try it with other accessories and choose the best combination. Sit, climb stairs, move in it. Wear it to a less important activity first, if possible, but allow time for stain removal should a mishap occur.

Avoid anything extreme, dramatic or attention attracting unless you allow yourself plenty of time to achieve perfection in the total look. Lapses in grooming, an extra 5 pounds, or not-quite-right accessories will make the spotlight an uncomfortable place to be.

The Rule of Fourteen. Women have found this to be a useful tool in controlling excess pattern/clutter/busyness. When completely dressed, stand before a full length mirror and count everything.

Give a point to each visible item of clothing. Now add an extra point for each patterned item worn, each accent color, each decorative trim, each piece of jewelry. Add extra points for colored or textured hose, for exposed handkerchiefs, for non-self belts and ornamental buttons. Be sure to count your handbag. And your hat, if worn. Contrasting trim and interesting hardware on a bag earns a total of three points instead of the one a simple bag would yield.

T-4s will wish to keep their score between nine and twelve, T-1s and T-2s between eleven and fourteen, and T-3s between twelve and sixteen. If your score is higher than it should be, remove an item or two to keep under the limit. If your count is too low, add something. You'll look far sharper with this kind of discipline.

Three magic steps.

1. Check each item you wear against your Type. Is it right for a T-2? a T-4?
2. Check your total look against your Type. Do you look like a T-4? a T-1?
3. Do you look like yourself and love it? If not, you need some additional information on figure disguise and display. And that just happens to come in the next chapter.

15

Disguise and Display

You began this book expecting to learn how best to dress. By now do you feel you've acquired two more balls than you can juggle? Sorry. It can't be helped. Many considerations enter into building a fine wardrobe. And, unfortunately, there's yet *another* ball to add to your collection before choosing clothes. Master it and you graduate to intelligent shopping.

This last, highly-important element is your *figure*. Stunning people *appear* to have NO figure faults. Not so. They have as many as you. But, they cleverly project an illusion of beauty that disguises their flaws and displays their assets.

Projecting beauty requires honesty. No blinders now. Unless you *recognize* your figure irregularities you can't hide them. Unless you know your good points, you can't showcase them.

Your tools for self-discovery will be accurate scales, a non-stretch, fabric tape measure, one strip of light cardboard measuring 1" x 10", a pencil and five photographs of YOU.

— FIVE PHOTOS —

Arrange for an amateur photographer to shoot black and white images of you. Stand in the shade if the day is bright, in the open if the sky is overcast. Select a plain background. Wear a bathing suit plus shoes with your most-often-worn heel height. These pictures won't be beautiful, but they'll be the most valuable *ugly* prints you'll ever own.

Stand, facing the camera with your hands at your sides yet slightly away from your torso. Feet should be parallel with weight evenly distributed. Look straight ahead. Have the photographer shoot at belt level, directly in front of you, filling the frame but not cropping your hair or your feet. *Click*.

Yes, you should *always* turn your torso for becoming pictures, but not this time. Beauty isn't our current object.

Turn completely around, back to the camera, for your second shot. Again, line up your feet, straighten your frame, look forward and have the camera at belt level. Hear the *click* behind you.

For your third picture, turn your side to the camera. Toes and head must point straight ahead; one shoulder, hip and ear toward the photographer. You'll hear the *click* from belt level.

The next two shots will prove invaluable when you get to the sections on cosmetics and hairstyling.

Wet your hair and comb it back from your face. Look straight into the camera. Lift your chin until your lower jaw is parallel to the ground. The frame should be filled with your face and head, the camera held at nose level. *Click*.

Last shot is a profile, so turn ninety degrees away from the camera. Again your head should fill the frame. *Click*.

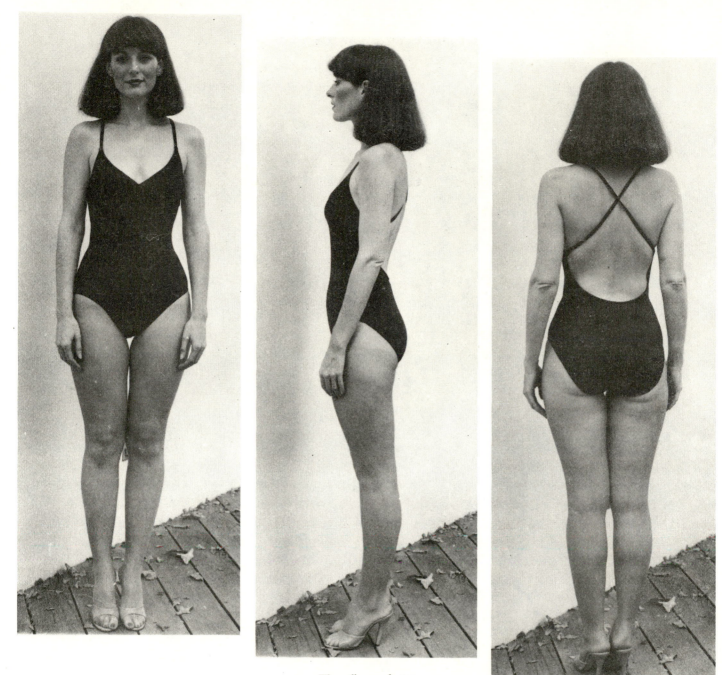

Three figure photos

Request an 8″ x 10″ print of each picture *plus the negatives.* You don't want to be blackmailed.

— WEIGHT CHECK —

While you wait for the film to be developed and printed, check your weight on accurate scales. Then hurry home and check it again on your own scales. Adjust yours to correspond with the scales in the doctor's office or wherever you found them. Keep your scales at this new setting.

First thing each morning, weigh yourself. Record your weight and the date on a pad near the scales and keep a running score. If your weight is constant and pleases you, omit the daily recordkeeping, but write today's weight and date in the PERSONAL RECORDS chart which follows.

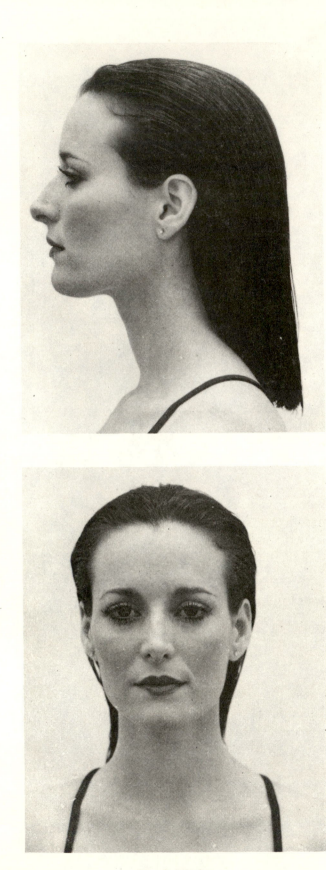

Two facial photos

Find your IDEAL weight on the height-/weight guide and record it in the last column of the Weight line in your PERSONAL RECORDS chart.

If you'd be heavier or lighter than you are, note each week's weight in the spaces provided, weighing always at the same time of day and same day of the week. You'll soon see progress.

— MEASUREMENT CHECK —

Use a fabric tape measure to establish your exact dimensions. Keep the tape snug but not tight. It should be parallel to the floor. Omit any bulk between you and the tape. Women should measure over bras, if they wear them, but not over girdles.

Measure your bust/chest at its fullest, waist at the slimmest, hip at the socket which joins leg to trunk, thigh just below the groin, calf at its fullest and ankle just above the ankle bone. Measure your upper arm midway between elbow and shoulderpoint, wrist just above the wristbone. Record all measurements on page 88, first column.

Height/Weight Guide For Women

Height*	Small Frame (Pounds)	Medium Frame (Pounds)	Large Frame (Pounds)
6'0 "	138-148	144-159	153-173
5'11"	134-144	140-155	149-168
5'10"	130-140	136-151	145-163
5'9 "	126-135	132-147	141-158
5'8 "	121-131	128-143	137-154
5'7 "	118-127	124-139	133-150
5'6 "	114-123	120-135	129-146
5'5 "	111-119	116-130	125-142
5'4 "	108-116	113-126	121-138
5'3 "	105-113	110-122	118-134
5'2 "	102-110	107-119	115-131
5'1 "	99-107	104-116	112-128
5'0 "	96-104	101-113	109-125
4'11"	94-101	98-110	106-122
4'10"	92-98	96-107	104-119

Note: For women between 18 and 25, subtract one pound for each year under 25.
*With shoes with two-inch heels.
Source: Boehringer Ingelheim, Ltd., Elmsford, N.Y. 10523

Height/Weight Guide For Men

Height*	Small Frame (Pounds)	Medium Frame (Pounds)	Large Frame (Pounds)
6'4 "	164-175	172-190	182-204
6'3 "	160-171	167-185	178-199
6'2 "	156-167	162-180	173-194
6'1 "	152-162	158-175	168-189
6'0 "	148-158	154-170	164-184
5'11"	144-154	150-165	159-179
5'10"	140-150	146-160	155-174
5'9 "	136-145	142-156	151-170
5'8 "	132-141	138-152	147-166
5'7 "	128-137	134-147	142-161
5'6 "	124-133	130-143	138-156
5'5 "	121-129	127-139	135-152
5'4 "	118-126	124-136	132-148
5'3 "	115-123	121-133	129-144
5'2 "	112-120	118-129	126-141

*With shoes with one-inch heels.
Source: Boehringer Ingelheim, Ltd., Elmsford, N.Y. 10523

— PERSONAL RECORDS —

date									ideal
*Weight									
*Measurements									
bust/chest									
waist									
hips									
upper thigh									
knee									
calf									
ankle									
upper arm									
wrist									

Visual Proportions in Head Lengths	My HL	Average HL	
		her	him
*Horizontal			
shoulders		1 1/2	2
bust/chest		1 1/4	1 1/4+
waist		1-	1+
hips		1 1/2+	1 1/4
thighs (both together)		1 1/2	1 1/4
Vertical			
top of skull to bust/chest		2	2
top of skull to waist		2 2/3	2 2/3
top of skull to hip		3 3/4	3 2/3
top of skull to thigh		4 1/4	4 1/2
top of skull to knee		5 1/2	5 1/2
top of skull to calf		5 2/3	5 5/6
top of skull to ankle		6 3/4	7
top of skull to soles of shoes		7 1/2	7 1/2

*May be changed via diet and exercise.

88

— FIGURE IRREGULARITIES —

(*my* problems are underlined)

head—large, small, forward

neck—long, short, thick, thin, dowager's hump, wrinkled

back—broad, narrow

shoulders—wide, narrow, square, sloping, forward curving, one high

arms—long, short, heavy, thin, elbow above/below center

bust—large, flat, high, low, uneven sides

chest—flat, narrow, barrel, pidgeon-breasted

waist—thick, thin, wide, high, low

abdomen—prominent

hips—square, straight, wide, narrow, one high

buttocks—prominent, flat, high, low

thighs—long, short, thick, thin, too close, too distant

knees—large, small, wide, narrow, too far apart

calves—thick, thin, no-curve

lower legs—long, short, thick, thin

ankles—thick, thin, irregular

feet—long, short, thin, thick, awkward

wrists—thin, thick, bony

hands—long, short, thick, thin, veined

fingers—long, short, thick, thin, irregular

My BEST features are:_____

_____

_____

— VISUAL PROPORTIONS CHECK —

When your photos return, take out the full-figure front view. With it you'll need a pencil and the straight strip of cardboard. This procedure can furnish information not availble from scales and measurements.

Place one narrow edge of the cardboard strip at the top of your photographed head, one side cutting your body in half. Mark the strip at a point level with the bottom of your chin. Now slip the cardboard upwards until the *mark* is at the top of your head and again place a line on the edge level with the bottom of your chin. Repeat until you've marked the entire length of cardboard.

Subdivide the first marked segment into halves, quarters and eighths, as a standard ruler is subdivided.

You've just made a ruler that measures *head-lengths* instead of inches. It's accurate only for you and with this one photograph.

Now measure your shoulder width on the photo with your new ruler. Record that number in the *My HL* (My Head-Lengths) column. Note the average woman's shoulders measures 1 1/2 HL while the average man's measure two HL.

Complete the rest of the *My HL* column by measuring your image on the photograph and recording your numbers of Head Lengths. those with unusually large or small heads in relation to their bodies will find their numbers differing from those given in the Average HL column. If this is your problem, don't worry. Merely underline "large" or "small" head under Figure Irregularities.

— PERSONAL EVALUATION —

What do all the figures mean? They indicate *where you differ from the norm.* And since the most gorgeous people around have areas in which they also differ, you shouldn't mind joining them and the rest of the human race.

Place a check (✔) in the margin next to any line of your Personal Record that shows a variance.

You can easily note whether you weigh less or more than the ideal for your bone structure, but the bust/chest/waist/hip measurements have no such ideal listing. That's right. They are included for you to record today's dimensions. When you retake those measurements you'll see change and be faced with the direction of the change—whether toward smaller or larger.

Additional proportions may help in your figure assessment. The hipline divides the normal figure in half. The ideal bustline is midway between shoulder and waist. Knees subdivide legs into two equal parts, as elbows divide arms. Women's elbows reach their waists and wrists touch their hips. Men's elbows and wrists reach lower on their torsos.

Look at your front, back and sideview photos. They'll help you fill-out your Figure Irregularities section. If you see no assets in the pictures, dress up, do your hair and look for your best features in the mirror. Or you can ask a friend to list your best features.

— ILLUSION —

To have an "illusion of beauty":

Play-up, spotlight, enhance your good features.

Disguise your poor features.

Emphasize by revealing, by close fit, or by accenting with the unexpected: a bright color, a rough texture, patterned design, shiny surface, or contrast of dark/light, smooth/rough, dull/shiny, plain/print.

Most common place for emphasis is your *face*. Unless your waist is tiny, legs are lissome, hands or feet are superb, chest hair is masterful or decolleté fetching, keep all attention on your face.

Be cautious of emphasizing tiny feet if legs and ankles aren't equally fine, or if feet are too small for your height and torso. Don't emphasize a tiny waist if by doing so your bust looms forward like a pigeon's. Be aware of overall effect.

Repeat only *flattering* lines.

Deemphasize with limited contrast and darker, smoother, duller, plainer choices. Mask, cover up, break up the area, or direct attention elsewhere.

When hips are wide and shoulders narrow, build-out your upper silhouette with horizontal lines like yokes, shoulder detailing, shoulder pads, and full-topped sleeves. Keep your lower section as simple, dark, dull and smooth as possible.

When an area is broader than you wish, subdivide it with vertical lines. The too-wide shoulders are best narrowed with vertical seaming, lapels, V or U necklines and chains or jewelry. Sleeves need a smooth cap to lessen apparent width.

Too-short areas can be visually elongated with vertical lines, too-long areas visually shortened when horizontal lines break up their length.

For skillful disguise of most common problems . . .

CHOOSE	AVOID

Too Tall?

soft lines; long jackets; tunics; wide collars and belts; medium-sized prints; contrasting colors; horizontal details	severely tailored or fussy items; skimpy cuts; short cuffs and hems; clingy fabrics; vertical details; stripes

Too Short?

simple lines and details; one color ensembles; vertical lines; narrow, matching belts; boleros; high waist styles	heavy or large details; boxy or long jackets; wide belts; horizontal lines; anything full or wide.

Too Thin?

bulky or stiff fabrics; light colors; patterns; contrasting colors; covered necklines	clingy tight, slim, straight lines; bareness; vertical details

Too Heavy?

dark or neutral colors; small patterns; dull finishes; one-color outfits; vertical details; self-belts; covered look; slightly-long pants, slightly-short longsleeves	large areas of bold color; plaid, shiny, heavy, bulky, stiff or clingy fabrics; wide or contrast belts; anything skimpy; too short a pant; too long a sleeve

Full Bosom?

vertical details; loosely fit, wrap styles; V or scoop necklines; simpler and darker tops; flared skirts; Chanel suits	shiny, heavy, bulky tops; pockets; double-breasted styles; round, bateau, high necklines; wide belts; tight skirts; puffed or cap sleeves

Full Hips?

dark pants with light shirt or jacket; flared skirts; short jackets	bright, print, shiny or flimsy fabric; below waist trims; pleats; gathers; long jackets

CHOOSE	AVOID

Over-Waistline Bulge?

tunics; overblouses; loose fit; longline bra or a one-piece foundation	tight, wide, contrasting belts; too-tight pants or skirts; strained-buttonhole look

Large Abdomen?

unpressed side pleats; broad shoulder lines; side-draped or flared skirts	center buttons or trim; sloping shoulder lines gored, tight or bouffant skirts

Bra Bulge?

wider backed, larger sized bra; crisp, opaque tops; back yokes	bra too small or narrow; low-cut styles; slinky or see-through tops

Long Waisted?

wide waistbands and belts; straight belts; short jackets; high-waisted pants and skirts; empire lines	narrow belts or waistless styles; low-waisted effects; vertical design in tops

Short Waisted?

single color costumes; long overblouses; no-waistband pants and skirts; hip-huggers; narrow, self and contour belts	contrast between upper and lower torso; boleros and short vests; wide waistbands or belts; empire effects

Short Neck?

open, V and T-shirt neck-lines; short hair; pendants	turtlenecks; bulky collars; long, full hair; chokers

Long Neck?

turtles, high necklines; stand-up collars; scarves; long hair hanging free	V or scooped necklines; strapless styles; short or upswept hair; long beads or chains

CHOOSE	AVOID

Heavy Arms?

well-cut sleeve; wide arm-hole; 3/4 length sleeve	sleeveless or short sleeves; tightly fitted sleeves

Thin Arms?

loose sleeves; wide cuffs;	sleeveless and short-sleeved styles; tightly fitted sleeves

Long Arms?

sleeves full and slightly long	short, narrow sleeves and 3/4 and 7/8 lengths

Short Arms?

sleeveless, narrow, slightly-short long sleeves 3/4 and 7/8 lengths	full sleeves, long cuffs, short and cap styles

And for your last "tool" in selecting camouflage, consider:

— USING YOUR "PHOTO DOLL" —

Look through current fashion magazines and select three potentially becoming styles. Assemble your figure photos, a pencil and a few sheets of tracing paper.

Lay one sheet of tracing paper over your front-view photograph and sketch the design you see in the magazine, or the patternbook (if you sew). Sketch the neckline, sleeves, waist, pant, whatever. Trace your hair, face, arms, legs. You'll note a difference between your proportions and the model's, but that's expected.

Sketch a second then a third style. Compare the three sketches. Which is the most becoming to you? Which best disguises your handicaps, displays your assets? See page 94.

Sketch your best style in both side and back views. Does it still pass the test? If so, head for the stores to try on that style and let a mirror reinforce your knowledge. Only then do you consider buying or making this style in a color, fabric and fit that meets your wardrobe requirements, climate and budget. Be highly critical. Expect a lot from your clothes.

Fashionable skirt lengths vary seasonally so always try new styles and lengths on your Photo Doll before adjusting those you own. Most pleasing proportion remains 1/3 leg and 2/3 costume. It's something to remember.

The more you work with disguise and display techniques, the better you'll become at spotlighting and camouflage. But, you'll soon realize changing your imperfections is easier than constantly disguising them. This leads us to our next chapter where *Recontouring* is the subject.

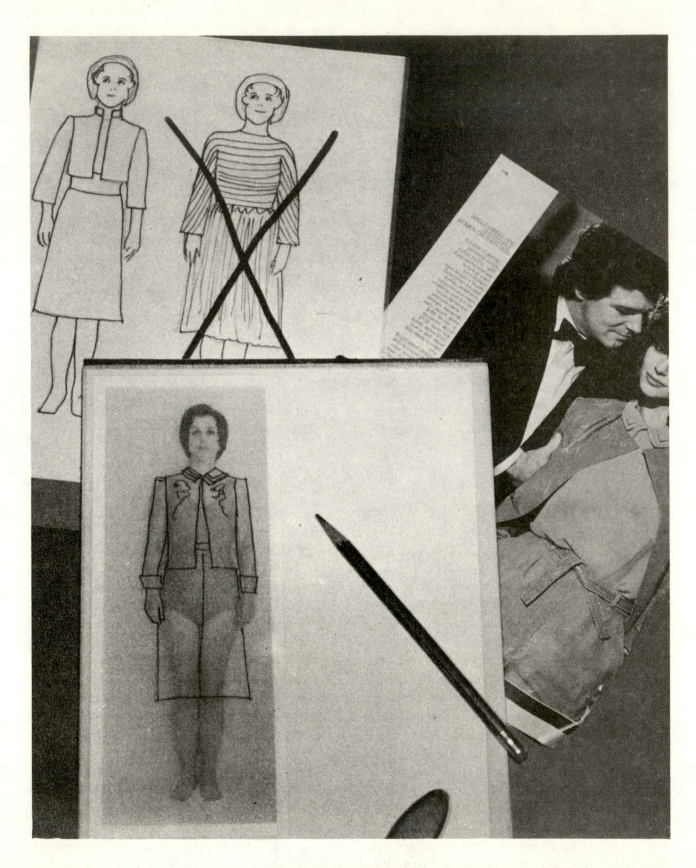

Using your "Photo Doll"

94

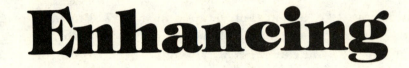
Enhancing

16

Your Body

Would you like an instant ten-pound weight loss? Of course it's impossible without drastic surgery, but you can *apparently* weigh ten pounds less by standing tall. Poor posture adds bulk to your torso. An erect body dramatically slims.

— POSTURE —

Pull out your figure photos and check your posture in profile. Does a straight-edge dividing your ear and your ankle also halve your torso? It should. On your front and back photos are shoulders level, hips? They should be, but if they aren't correction is possible.

Improved posture comes with practice. Standing tall enhances your health, proportions, and clothing; builds your self-esteem; increases your comfort; and, incidentally, cuts an average of one-inch from your waist measurement.

To Improve Your Posture:
1. Stand as if drawn upward by a cord connected to the top of your head. You're a marionette with your chin parallel to the floor.
2. Relax your shoulders and let your arms and hands hang limply.
3. Lift your chest, as with a deep breath.
4. Lift your waist up and away from your hips.
5. Flatten your back, drawing hips down and under the body, straightening your spine.
6. Keep knees and feet together, knees slightly bent and weight on the balls of your feet.

7. Practice upright posture when you arise each morning, each time you step before a mirror, pause at a stoplight, wait for an elevator, whenever you sit down, and whenever you feel tired or ache.

The more you practice, the more natural aligned posture becomes. Someday you'll be complimented on how well you look, how straight you stand. You'll usually decrease one clothing size when poor posture has flown.

If your body tips sideways, one shoulder or hip high or low, consider switching to the other hand for carrying your handbag, the other hip for hefting the baby or the opposite side for the activities of your job. By using both sides equally, symmetry can be regained.

A most helpful tool for improving posture is Marjorie Craig's classic *21 Day Shape-up Program for Men and Women*. Ms. Craig has a section on posture-improving exercises which work. Do them, along with her other prescribed daily exercises, for three weeks, and you'll be picking up compliments on your weight-loss even if you haven't lost an ounce. As a bonus, these exercises are quiet and non-vigorous. They're perfect beginning exercises for those unused to physical activity and for those wishing a daily meditating/communing time.

— EXERCISE —

But quiet exercises aren't enough. The President's Council on Physical Fitness and Sports states, "Without cardiopulmonary fitness you are not fit." Any exercise program which fails to vigorously involve your heart and lungs over a period of time fails as your sole form of exercise. Activities which tone or build muscles, add limberness and strength yet fail to adequately exercise the heart and lungs include yoga, isometrics (muscles teamed against other muscles or an unmoveable object), and most isokinetics (muscles against machines or weights.)

Why exercise vigorously? It's tiring, sweaty, achy business which ruins hairdos and eats up your time. Sitting or lying feels far more comfortable and reasonable. But vigorous exercise:

Trims and streamlines your figure. Well-exercised muscles have tone, strength and better support your body. Waist, hips, buttocks and thighs are particularly benefited.

Improves your circulation and skin-tone. Does "rosy with health" describe your skin-tone? A number of people have dramatically recovered from chronic skin eruptions as soon as they began a regular jogging program.

Keeps you looking young. The youngest, healthiest-appearing older men and women are those who regularly and actively exercise. Those who sit, *wither.*

Prolongs life. Diseases of the heart, veins, lungs and intestines come with sedentary lifestyles. Regular, sustained physical activity heals and rebuilds, returning health.

Increases energy, enthusiasm and sexual appetite. A toned body readily responds to stimuli.

Decreases stress and anxiety. Life's steadily increasing pressures are killing. Vigorous exercise is a fine antidote.

Relaxes and promotes sleep better than a tranquilizer.

Aids regularity. Physical activity stimulates the intestines and eliminates constipation.

Cuts out potential calories. Hurries food through the intestines and shortens absorption time.

Burns extra calories. Metabolism, the rate at which you burn oxygen (and thus food, which is your fuel), is elevated both during the activity and for several hours thereafter.

Depresses appetite by raising your blood sugar for a significant length of time.

Raises your calorie allowance. By increasing body mass (bone and muscle) your caloric needs increase. Thus you lose weight faster or you can eat more without gaining. Ideally, men have 10-15 percent body fat, women 15-25 percent. Fat is maintained by very few calories. In other words an obese person may have a caloric requirement of a 100 pounder although weighing 250 pounds. No wonder only 2 percent of dieters sustain a permanent weight loss with diet alone.

Increases bone densities. Those who live sedentary lives have a slow calcium drain, whereas active persons build calcium into their most-used bones.

Burns off triglycerides, preventing gout and improving your blood.

Helps prevent heart disease. 700,000 Americans die each year from hearts that stop pumping. During each minute of your life, your heart beats at least 70-72 times, pumping just over 5 quarts of blood. There's no rest for your heart. Each day has 1,440 minutes or more than 100,000 heartbeats.

To protect this precious organ consider sustained exercise. The long-distance runner's heart at rest beats approximately 30-35 times a minute, *half* what yours beats. These beats are deeper than yours, equally effective, but the slowness allows the heart to rest between beats. The runner's heart only works half as hard.

— BEFORE YOU EXERCISE —

Have a thorough physical. Any change in lifestyle puts a temporary strain upon your system. Have the doctor's okay before you buy running shoes. An annual checkup is excellent insurance, anyway.

Read Dr. Kenneth H. Cooper's paperback best sellers, *Aerobics* and *Aerobics for Women.* Absorb what he says. You'll be encouraged to work up to fitness. Keep track of your points!

Choose your activity. Best exercise is that which gets your heart to beating strongly and keeps it working steadily over a period of time. Read a book about your chosen sport/activity before you begin. Tips on how to start, needed equipment, and what to avoid should prove invaluable.

— EXERCISES —

Walking: one of the easiest motions for the previously inactive. You were designed for walking. Walk briskly, don't stroll, increase your distance regularly. Work toward a fifteen minute mile.

Jogging: cheapest, quickest, most efficient way to get into shape. Don't give up on your first few attempts. That first quarter-mile stays the hardest for most joggers.

Cycling: the best possible energy-saving activity. This fast, effective people-propeller trims the mid-to-lower torso and ups the heartrate—just what the doctor orders, most literally. If weather is foul or you can't get outside, consider a stationary bicycle in front of the television. Set a timer and pump away for an ever increasing time or tension, or both.

Swimming: elongates muscles, tones, and functions admirably as an aerobic exercise if you swim far and fast enough to count. Lucky, those with the use of a pool!

Rope Skipping: another quick, inexpensive means to health improvement. Boredom can be a problem, so plan ahead and jump yourself into shape.

Roller Skating: newest sport for grown-ups has changed completely from the skate-keyed metal strap-ons in which you once circled the block. Technology has produced a miracle of quietness and efficiency. Try the new skates at a rink. You may want to purchase a pair and roller-skate your way to shape in your own neighborhood.

Ice Skating: is a beautiful and graceful sport which earns aerobic points all the time you actually skate. If you have regular access to a rink, lucky you.

Dancing: is wonderful exercise, provided you *dance*, not just sway in each other's arms or watch from the sidelines. Best dances have active motions, naturally. Square dancing, folk dancing and disco can all give a fine workout, provided you have room to move. Ballroom dancing depends upon your ability. Fred Astaire earned his aerobic points.

Aerobic Dance: is a group exercise program developed by California choreographer, Jackie Sorenson, for women. Picture yourself in a chorus line dancing to disco, Latin or classical melodies, square-dancing without a partner, instructor calling each movement before you make it and showing you how. A heart monitoring program is built into the hour-long classes. Try it. You'll like it!

Tennis Singles: demands ability and a good opponent if you'd gain true exercise. You should be constantly running, shifting, stroking, not standing at ease while the inefficient player picks up the ball.

Water Skiing: counts for the time you're up on the skis.

Snow Skiing: uses different muscles but even downhill skiing can count while you're moving but not while you rest on the hill or stand in lift lines.

Cross-country Skiing: is the very best form of skiing for a full workout.

Handball/Squash/Volleyball/Basketball/Football: can all be counted toward your aerobic points if the game is fastpaced, you have proficiency, and you count only the time you actually play.

Sports vary in aerobic benefit. Golf doesn't count as a heartbeat raiser nor does target archery or tennis doubles even though they are far better than a shaded hammock. Bowling may be fun, but it doesn't raise your heartbeat over a sustained period.

If you're currently sedentary, think of all the painless ways you can add activity to your life. Sitting is better than lying-down and standing better than sitting, provided you move as you sit or stand. A rocking chair is better than a lounge chair. When you sit or stand still, your heart works hard to pump the blood up from your toes to your chest. When you move about, muscles assist the heart with its pumping.

If you get off the elevator one or more stops below your floor and climb that extra flight or two or three daily, you'll see improvement in your legs, your wind, and your circulatory system. If you park the car farther from work, you'll likely save money and have the added physical advantages that walking supplies. If you make large motions instead of tiny ones when bending, making beds, reaching, you're helping your system.

After a few weeks of adding easy motion to your schedule, do consider adding an aerobic activity. It pays valuable dividends. You'll see positive results within four to six weeks of regular, three to five times a week, workouts. Plan on continuing your exercise program for as long as you live. One's loss of muscle tone begins within the first month of inactivity.

— DIET —

Have you waited breathlessly for the word DIET? Recontouring can most definitely be speeded up by changing your caloric consumption (the quantity and kind of food you eat). But background information comes first.

Calories measure energy. You take-in calories with your food and drink. You use-up calories by being alive and through activity.

Calories count. When you eat more calories than your body burns you gain weight. When you eat fewer calories than your body burns you lose weight.

Four types of food and beverages contain calories.

1. *Protein* foods like meat, fish, poultry, eggs, milk and cheese.
2. *Carbohydrate* foods like bread, cereal, pasta, fruit, vegetables, sugar, syrup and candy.
3. *Fat* foods like butter, mayonnaise, sour cream, gravy, chocolate and rich pastries.
4. *Alcoholic beverages* like scotch, bourbon, gin, rum, wine and beer.

Fat foods contain more than twice as many calories as do proteins, carbohydrates or alcohol. Fat provides nine calories for each gram consumed while carbohydrate, protein, and alcohol only provide four calories per gram. A gram is a unit of weight.

A pound of body weight is equal to 3500 calories. To lose one pound you must eat 3500 calories fewer than your body burns. To gain, you must consume that amount more. Fortunately, loss or gain can be spread over a period of time. Eliminating two pats of butter each day will drop your weight one pound a week, if all else is held constant.

Each year you require fewer calories, for with age bodies become more efficient. This means eliminating, permanently, one item from your diet each year in order to keep your optimum weight.

Diet drugs are dangerous. Lowering your weight with drugs can destroy health yet not affect your long-term eating patterns. Weight comes right back.

Permanent weight loss or gain comes by permanently changing our eating and exercise patterns. Temporary gains or losses merely destroy the fit of your clothes and often your health.

Before you choose a diet read a late edition of Theodore Berland and the Editors of Consumer Guide's *Rating the Diets*. The diets you'll be considering are listed and rated.

Successful dieting is only possible when you feel comfortable with yourself. You need positive "strokes," as does everyone. Find support through faith in God, love of a friend, hypnosis, behavior modification, or diet groups like Weight Watchers and Overeaters Anonymous. Motivation also comes through the pleasure of your reflected image in Becoming Colors and an attractive wardrobe. You *can* add beauty of contour to your other pluses.

Total beauty is often blocked by just one thing. That's the subject of the next chapter, Personal Care, another way of saying GROOMING.

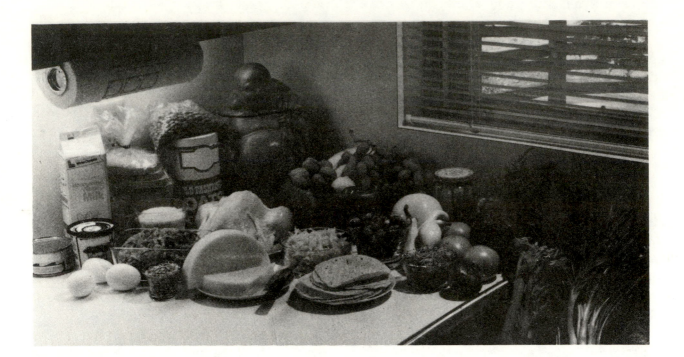

Beauty Foods
1. Meat/fish/poultry/eggs/beans for protein
2. Milk/cheese/yogurt for calcium & protein
3. Cereal/bread/seeds/nuts for vitamins/minerals
4. Fruits/vegetables for roughage/vitamins/minerals

17

Your Person

Your ideal Beauty will differ from everyone else's, but all will share one trait. The beautiful, whether male or female, dark or fair, young or old, will be *well-groomed*. Any breach of grooming eliminates even the most perfectly proportioned face and figure from the winner's circle.

Lest *you* fall victim to lapses in personal hygiene, a checklist is supplied.

— GROOMING CHECKLIST —

Daily
shampoo (optional)
bath or shower
facial hair removal (men)
deodorant
dental care
facial care
hand care
glasses cleaned
fresh clothing
full length mirror check
adequate sleep

Weekly
shampoo & condition
eyebrows checked
body hair removed (women)
"thinning" skin
manicure
pedicure
elbows and heels
shoes shined
purse cleaned
jewelry cleaned
massage (if you can manage it)

Weekly grooming sessions should be as much a part of your schedule as weekly tennis or bridge dates. Plan a special time each week for pampering yourself. You're worth it! But now to specifics.

— BATHING —

Showers aren't masculine and baths feminine; rather, showers stimulate and baths soothe.

Choose a shower for quick cleaning, instant energy, increased circulation, and stimulated skin. Try washing with warm water and soap, rinsing in a tepid stream and finishing with cool. A hard spray stimulates the skin, but only the most gentle, tepid spray should ever touch hair or face. Both are delicate and need protection.

To alleviate sore muscles, direct a warm stream of water over the painful area for three minutes.

Before you leave a stall shower, squeegee walls and door. (This will quickly lessen humidity and housekeeping chores.) Then, buff yourself dry with a thick, terry towel.

Choose a bath when you have time and

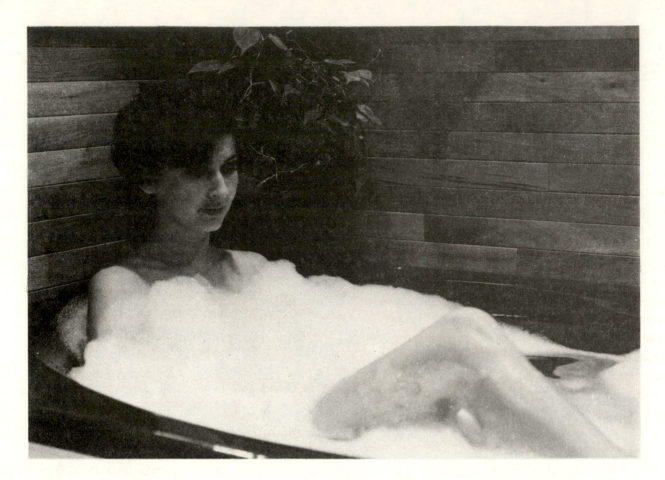

T-4 bathing

wish a soothing release from soil, tension, fatigue, heat or cold.

Step into the luxury of deep, warm water. Soften your bath with bubbles, oil, gel, beads or salts. Epson salts, baking soda or a cheesecloth-wrapped handful of regular oatmeal are less exotic but have their own charms.

When January chilled, have your bath warmer than your body temperature, perhaps 102°F. If July sweltering, choose a cooler than body temp, such as 92°F. Lie back, close your eyes and let worries float away.

Consider a loofah a necessity for bath or shower. It's a strange, sponge-like gourd that softens and swells in water yet retains sufficient crispness to gently abrade the outer layers from your skin. This "thins" your skin, decreases the size of your pores, and improves your circulation. Use at least once a week over your entire body.

— HAIR REMOVAL —

Unsightly hair must either go under wraps or go away. It is never seen on the well-groomed. How do you remove this hair without harming your skin? Men have basically two options for facial hair removal: *shaving wet* with a sharp blade or *shaving dry* with an electric shaver. Women may adapt the same techniques for de-hairing legs, but they have additional options.

Shaving Wet requires hair to be soft and weak, skin to be lubricated. Begin by thoroughly soaking, soaping and rinsing your face/legs and then splashing repeatedly with warm water. Apply a moisturizer to lock in the wetness. Then, if your skin is sensitive or dry, apply a brushless shaving cream. If your skin is oily, choose a foamy type.

Use a clean, sharp blade. Assure cleanliness by rinsing the razor under running water, pouring alcohol over the blade then rinsing again. Change blades at least weekly for sharpness. And, *stroke the way the hair grows, not against it.* Admittedly, you'll not get as close a shave going with your hair's growth, but you'll cut down on skin irritation. Men shave chin and upper lip last to allow the longest softening time.

Rinse thoroughly, again and again, to remove all traces of soap. Then moisturize. A styptic pencil (sold in drugstores) will stop bleeding should you nick yourself.

Shaving Dry requires hairs to be at their driest and stiffest. Both moisture and lubricants, which can protect your face from the electric razor, make shaving more difficult. What to do? Use a good pre-electric shave preparation. It is designed to evaporate quickly, leaving your beard stiff and your skin protected. Again, stroke with the hair, not against it. Shave gently. Clean your shaver, after each use, with the small brush provided by the manufacturer.

Now, wash with soap and water then rinse again and again. You aren't finished until you moisturize. If you have acne or severe blemishes check with your dermatologist about moisturizing.

Men with dark hair and fair skin may have to shave *twice* a day to escape "five-o'clock shadow." It's unfortunate, but T-4s can't have *everything*. Alternatives might be to grow beards or to thin the beard area with electrolysis.

Options other than shaving include: electrolysis, depilatation, waxing, tweezing and bleaching.

Electrolysis is more expensive and ultimately permanent. Hair is killed by cauterization when a slight electric current is passed to the bottom of each follicle via a thin needle. Warmth or tingling are the general sensations. Expect to follow directions such as not scratching or rubbing treated areas, applying icepacks when indicated, and returning for treatment when new hairs become tweezable.

First consultations with an electrologist are usually free and treatments are set-up by time, not numbers of hairs. Return visits are necessary since 20 percent of body hair is dormant at any one time, and tough hair or deformed hairshafts often require more than one treatment.

Electrolysis is superb for reshaping brows, hairlines, necklines, thinning beards, shortening sideburns and removing facial hair. Consider having a beauty authority shape your brows and hairline *temporarily* before you have an electrologist shape them permanently. Having a permanently *bad* browline isn't much improvement, if any, over a hairy one. Never let anyone treat your inside nose or ears for the same reason that you don't tweeze hairs that reside there—infection. All other body areas respond well to electrolysis.

Not all states register electrologists, so seek a competent one who's a member of a related professional organization and recommended by friends or doctor.

Depilatories, like good shavers, are fast and easy. They work chemically by dissolving the hair shaft at the skinline. This provides the advantage of a somewhat slower regrowth but the disadvantage of possibly irritating tender skin. Follow manufacturer's directions, *exactly*.

Waxing lasts two to six weeks and regrowth is soft, but it's difficult to do by oneself and somewhat expensive. Waxing works mechanically by trapping hairs in a substance which hardens around them. When the substance is quickly pulled away from the area, the hair comes away, too, as if it were tweezed.

Tweezing works best for stray or wild hairs. Clean tweezers in alcohol then rinse in water before using. If you're tweezing many hairs, first chill the area with a washcloth wrapped icecube. Then, pull as the hair grows. Apply alcohol to the treated area, rinse with water, and moisturize.

NEVER TWEEZE HAIRS FROM YOUR NOSE OR EARS. Horrible infections lie in wait for those making this mistake. Clip visible hairs from nose and ears each week during your weekly grooming time.

Both waxing and tweezing tend to distort hair follicles, making later electrolysis more difficult.

Bleaching is best for fine hairs which only show because of their darkness. Follow product directions *exactly*.

Individuals are excessively hairy for a variety of reasons: heredity; glandular disturbances; systemic changes such as puberty, menopause or senescence; and irritation as from long incarceration in a cast. You may have a problem, but it needn't be a permanent one.

Unsightly hair includes: visible facial hair, hair growing from moles, ears, noses, straying eyebrows, wild hairs in eyebrows (pull or clip them) and, for women, hairy faces, arms, underarms, thighs, legs, hands and feet. The hirsute female has been admired in other eras and cultures, but not this one.

— DEODORANTS —

A bath or shower and fresh clothing, daily, helps check body odor, but a good deodorant or antiperspirant adds further insurance against offending.

Choose a deodorant when you wish to control odor but amount of perspiration isn't a problem.

Choose an antiperspirant if you wish to check both wetness and odor.

You have a choice of cream, liquid, stick, spray, pad, rub-on and roll-on wet or dry products from as many different manufacturers. As with all personal products, experiment until you find one that works well for you.

Whatever form you use, apply it night and morning to clean, dry skin. Apply in a generous circle, covering the entire underarm area. If excess perspiration persists, wear dress shields and see your dermatologist for a prescription to control it.

Deodorant powder on your feet and in shoes, stockings, girdles and bras will absorb moisture and increase your protection. A special deodorant can be used on menstrual pads, but tampons, being internal, are even better protection from monthly odor. Change tampons and/or pads every three hours.

Douching and vaginal deodorants should be avoided unless prescribed by your doctor. Keep deodorant and anti-bacterial soaps away from vaginal areas. A moderate vaginal discharge is normal. See your gynecologist if your discharge is copious, smells unpleasant, causes itching or irritates your skin.

— DENTAL CARE —

Sparkling teeth, healthy gums and pleasant breath are infinitely appealing and come with a squeaky-clean mouth. But to reach "squeaky clean" you must first recognize the villains, plaque and tartar.

Plaque, a revolting, gluey blend of saliva, food particles and bacteria coats teeth and gums each time you eat. Within 24 hours plaque ferments to become an acid which destroys tooth enamel, infects gums and erodes the tissue and bone structure which support teeth.

When plaque's bacteria die, they begin calcifying and become a hard, visible film called *tartar*. Tartar irritates your gums, causing them to bleed and to recede. Noticed any "pink toothbrush" lately? Tartar is usually the cause. And it, unfortunately, can only be removed by your dentist.

Do you wonder that 95 percent of Americans have some kind of tooth problem and over 25 million are toothless?

But doesn't brushing control plaque buildup? Not entirely. Casual brushing removes about 20 percent of the plaque that is present. Brushing isn't enough. But plaque *can* be controlled. Here's how:

1. *Limit your intake of simple sugars and starches, for plaque thrives on them. But should you succumb to temptation—* brush *immediately*. Timing is important. If you can't brush, rinse with water.
2. *Floss daily with unwaxed dental floss.* To floss:
   a- Cut 18-inches of floss and wrap most of its length around the middle finger.

Wrap the opposite end around the middle finger of your other hand.

b- Consider your mouth to be in four parts: upper right, upper left, lower right, lower left.

c- Using the thumbs for the upper and index fingers for the lower, floss between all teeth in each section, unwinding floss from one hand and winding-up on the other, keeping a fresh area between your fingers.

d- Floss by gently working strand between teeth then rubbing it up and down on the sides of both adjoining teeth.

e- Now rinse your mouth vigorously with cool water.

3. *Brush your teeth* this way:

a- Alternate *two* toothbrushes, for best results

b- Replace brushes every three-four months as a new brush removes three-four times the plaque as an old one.

c- Choose *soft* bristles with a flat brushing surface.

d- Brush thoroughly at least once each day, preferably at night, or after every meal and sweet snack.

e- Use fluoride toothpaste or, if not available, water.

f- Brush gently, removing germs from every brushable surface: gums, tooth fronts, backs, cutting surfaces and tongue.

g- Rinse thoroughly with water. Use a mouthwash if you like, but its effects are temporary. Properly cleaned teeth are your best breath sweeteners.

h- Rinse your toothbrush and store where air circulates.

4. *Test the effectiveness of your mouth cleaning* by chewing a "disclosing tablet" (available at your druggist). It temporarily dyes plaque a red or purple, indicating areas you've missed. Rebrush those areas.

5. *See your dentist every six months* to assure yourself the villains are kept in check, to clean your teeth of plaque and tartar, X-ray for cavities, and make repairs.

If your teeth don't meet properly, making it difficult to bite through celery, or if they're crooked and unattractive, ask your dentist for the name of a good orthodontist. The nearly-invisible new braces aren't solely for children, and capping and coating techniques constantly improve. But a word of caution—don't let anyone coat or cap your teeth with a tone of white that is lighter than the whites of your eyes or your own teeth. A beautiful TV actress/singer/dancer has capped teeth that flash brilliantly. Her eyes are lost. Being upstaged is bad, but by your teeth!

— ADEQUATE SLEEP —

Sleep uses one-third of our lives and is as vital to that life as food and water. It's highly prized by models and actors who earn their living by looking attractive, while others destroy both health and looks by ignoring sleep requirements. Don't let it happen to you. Sufficient sleep is *essential* to your looks.

Not everyone requires eight hours sleep nightly. Requirements vary from four to twelve hours, decreasing in amount as one ages. You know when you're getting enough sleep.

Having trouble sleeping? It's common, so here are a few cures for insomnia.

1. A *good* mattress is not a luxury; it's a necessity and should be your first furnishing investment.

2. Room temperature of 60° to 64° are best for sleeping, but a quiet fan can make higher temperatures tolerable.

3. Include bananas, figs, pineapple, nuts, meat, poultry or eggs in your evening meal and drink a small glass of vermouth, gingerale, red wine or milk before bed. All encourage drowsiness.

4. Avoid coffee, tea, cola, chocolate, sangria, chianti, sherry, champagne, aged cheese, yogurt, sour cream, avocados and fish at supper and afterwards. They're proven stimulants.

5. Bridge, a lively argument, exercise, or a violent television program are no-nos before retiring.
6. Take a lukewarm bath. Relax. Dust yourself with talc. Don clean, loose sleepwear (optional).
7. Slip into a clean, tautly-made bed at the same time each night.
8. Cultivate serenity. Pray or meditate, relinquishing the day. Good-night.

On the nights you're stimulated yet long to sleep, take two aspirin and relax with a dull book until you become sleepy. Read in a chair, not your bed. Bed's for *sleeping*. Avoid sleeping pills. They're addictive and dangerous.

— EMERGENCY STRATEGY —

Often when traveling, and sometimes at home, you face small problems related to grooming. Here are some equally small solutions.

Lint on your navy flannel? Make a "knuckle duster" by wrapping scotch or masking tape several times around one hand. Barely overlap the layers with sticky side *out*. Press this tape onto the lint-covered surface and "voila," it's gone.

Shoes need emergency polishing? Slip one foot out of its shoe and polish the toe of the other with your nyloned sole. Reverse.

Pantyhose drawer empty? Suds previously-worn ones quickly, rinse, then roll in a turkish towel while you shower. Complete the drying process with your hairdryer. (Buying pantyhose by the dozen generally eliminates this problem.)

Runs in your pantyhose? Cut off the leg with runs and match it to a similar pair with a missing leg. Put on both panties and you'll be ready to go.

Runs in the same leg? Eliminate the cause (rough toenail, splinter on chair) then turn one single-legged pantyhose inside out. Put it on, then put on the mate. Wear with closed-toed shoes so toe seam can't show.

Blouse pulls out or blouse hem or color shows through your skirt? Tuck the tail of your blouse *inside* your pantyhose. They'll stay securely and the hem imprint will be lessened or eliminated. If you try this with pants, always check your back pant waistband when you're seated to be certain pantyhose elastic isn't peeking out.

No lingerie laundry soap? Use shampoo.

Dusting powder getting low? Blend it with cornstarch. The combination will feel marvelous on your skin.

Where's the information you need about skin care, manicures and shampooing? It's in the next chapters. Read on.

18

Your Skin

Intelligent, well-built, personable, Bill should have had everything, but he sat, head in hands, moaning, "Why couldn't I just have clear skin? That doesn't seem too much to ask." Bill's skin was pitted from his long feud with acne, and current lesions were causing renewed distress. Was he forever doomed?

Over a several year period Karen's fair skin had become masked with a brown pigment. Doctors called it abnormal cells and said that neither dermabrasion nor chemical peel would help. The abnormality went too deep. Doctors insisted she must be, or have been, using the "pill." Karen insisted she had not. The thought that she might always wear such a mask was intolerable.

Penny never stayed home. She was on the tennis court, the golf course, or discoing at the club from dawn to drop-into-bedtime. She felt young and alive while exhausting everyone else with her inexhaustable energy. Her problem? Her figure was lithe, but her face and limbs resembled the rough cowhide which covered her father's expensive luggage. Was it too late for Penny to swap her weathered face for a younger one?

No. There were solutions for all.

Bill and Karen needed help with their hormones, a diet which balanced their acidity, vitamins, and repeated skin layerings.

Layering uses a natural organic substance to clean impurities and sebum from hair follicles and remove all dead surface cells. It isn't dermabrasion or chemcial peel. It can be repeated weekly. Their skin-care program was monitored by Jeneal® International, Skin Correction Centers.

Bill and Karen weren't instantly cured—it took time to build new, healthier skin—but now they look wonderful.

Penny shifted to indoor athletics, hats and sunscreens, a balanced-acid diet, and repeated layerings. Her skin improved more than she expected but less than she'd hoped.

Skin advertises your health—glowing and moist or blemished by dark circles, pimples, scars, brown spots, oil slicks or dry, rough areas. Is your skin lifeless? Look in the mirror. Do you like your skin? If you don't, consider changing it. To do so . . .

Upgrade Your General Health. Eat a balanced diet; drink lots of water; get plenty of rest, exercise and fresh air; enjoy uplifting sex; and spend a portion of each day doing something you *want* to do.

See Your Physician. Ask to have a blood count, your thyroid checked, and your capacity to burn oxygen measured. Deficiencies in these areas show on faces.

Women should also ask for a *Maturation Index* (taken at the time of their Pap smear and in the same manner). This sample may be obtained anytime by non-menstruating women, but otherwise it must be scheduled between the twelfth and fifteenth day after the start of menstruation. It clinically indicates estrogen levels. If your estrogen level is proven low, talk to your doctor about estrogen therapy. But make sure any estrogen you take is derived from natural sources. Chemical estrogen has produced negative side effects.

Balance Your pH. Jeri O'Neal, President of Jeneal's® International, states that 90 percent of all cosmetic skin disorders come from acid/alkaline imbalance. Test yourself. Buy *Nitrazine paper* from your local druggist or ask him to order it from his Squibb supplier. Place a 3/4″ piece on your tongue. Wet it with saliva, and quickly check the color against the accompanying chart. Yellow or gold is 4.5 acidity or lower. Darkest blue is 7.5 alkalinity or higher. Your goal should be a saliva that tests 6.0, avocado green. Test yourself 15-20 minutes after eating or drinking.

Your grandmother must have served acidic cranberry sauce with her alkaline turkey; applesauce with pork; and vinegar with spinach. You can too. But don't be mislead into thinking that citrus and other fruits are acidic. Their salts are alkaline.

Many foods will test acid before you consume them, but later turn your saliva alkaline. Those which remain acidic are apples, applesauce, apple juice (not apple cider), cranberries and cranberry juice, strawberries, pickles, vinegar and prepared foods which contain a high vinegar content, such as oil and vinegar dressings, marinades and sweet and sour sauce.

Proteins react as alkalines. These include meat, fish, poultry, eggs and dairy products. Yeast, artificial sweeteners, coffee, tea and colas, and the fruit not mentioned in the acidic group generally test alkaline.

Most breads, cereals and grains, potatoes, celery, watermelon and papaya are neutral.

You'll soon be identifying your body's requirements, "Orange or apple juice for breakfast?" without the need of the Nitrazine test.

Avoid problem foods. Skin flareups are often caused by chocolate, cocoa and caffein products such as cola, coffee and tea; seafoods such as shrimp, lobster, oysters and crab; iodized salt; some nerve and headache medications containing bromides; fried foods, ham, pork, bacon, nuts and peanut butter. Limit your intake of meats, especially those smoked; spicy sauces such as Worcestershire, chili and catsup; and most dairy products. Cottage cheese can be used in moderation and you can drink up to three glasses of skim milk daily.

Nicotine ages. If you want lovely skin, remove yourself from the presence of tobacco smoke, either yours or theirs. Smog also ages.

Protect your skin from sunlight. Most dangerous times and places to bare your skin include: exposure for more than a few moments; between 10 A.M. and 4 P.M.; during the summer months; at high elevations, as when skiing; near water or sand's reflective qualities; and near the equator.

Best protecters when you *must* be out are opaque, long-sleeved clothing; dark glasses; wide-brimmed hats; and a block-out lotion containing 5 percent PABA, paradicholorobenzine.

Be careful of sun when you're pregnant. Brunettes, in particular, are prone to brown facial spots at this time.

Never tan a new scar. Your scar will retain its tan long after your skin has faded to pale.

Today's sunburn is twenty-years-from-today's cancer or wrinkles. Lucky the man or woman with black ancestry. The melanine in their skin acts as a sun filter. The darker the skin, the more protection, thus the slower they burn or age.

A few months of bronzing oneself is more damaging and aging than 100 years of living. The protected skin areas of very old individuals are smooth and young. Only exposed skin weathers.

Wind, heat and cold are also enemies. Windblown snow and cozy fires are *both* murder to your skin. Avoid the wind which strips moisture from your face in an instant, cold which can actually burn your skin as does heat. Run from heatlamps, sunlamps, hot water, hot towels, facial saunas, ovens and fireplaces unless you keep your distance or are under doctor's orders. Skin loves the moderate zones.

Cleanse properly. Look for a daily skin cleanser that removes all surface film, is non-irritating, and can be removed easily. How does YOUR cleanser stack up?

Your best cleansing agent will be a fragrance-free, cream-free, deodorant-free *soap*. Dry or sensitive skins may be happier with a *rinseable cleanser*, but any skin cleanser should have low viscosity (flows freely from the container) in order to glide onto and off-of the skin without dragging or moving the skin.

Pat either soapy lather or lotion onto your skin. Rinse immediately and very thoroughly, twenty or thirty times. Cleansers must be completely removed. They're important for their purpose but, by nature, harsh. Water is kind.

Astringents, toners and fresheners are fine cleaning aids. Use them after rinsing or in place of a morning cleaning. *Nothing*, however, should replace your nighttime cleaning. It's imperative.

Astringents contain more alcohol than do toners and fresheners, and diluted alcohol is a desirable ingredient. But if your face burns or capillaries become visible, your astringent is too strong. To eliminate the problem, dilute your astringent with a few drops of distilled or mineral water, or try the gentler *toner* or even the gentlest *freshener*.

Test your cleansing aids with Nitrazine paper. A pH of 4.5 to 5.5 is perfect, for it corresponds with the pH of your skin. Yes, your interior and exterior are both acidic, but not to the same degree. Look for a 4.5 to 5.5 pH on all skin and hair products.

Moisturize promptly. Since proper cleansing removes the skin's natural protection and moisture along with the dirt, they need replacement instantly. Moisturizers seal the skin's surface, slow the evaporation of water, protect, lubricate, and *should be worn at all times*. Apply lightly over *still-wet* skin. Your entire body needs moisturizing.

Choose a light, thin moisturizer if you are young, the weather is warm, or it's to be used under makeup. Choose a thicker form for older skin, colder weather, and bedtime wear. Oil of Olay® and Night of Olay® are products worth trying.

Test your moisturizer with Nitrazine paper. If your moisturizer doesn't have a pH of 4.5 to 5.5 change to one that does. You can take your test tape with you while shopping and thus pre-test all products before you purchase them.

Avoid moisturizers with color, fragrance, hormones, vitamins, proteins, milk, honey, strawberries, eggs, seaweed or cucumbers. These add expense, not effectiveness.

Men need moisturizers as much as women and, wisely, many are already using them.

Thin your skin weekly. Pores are tiny when skin is new and thin, but they become large when skin thickens with unsluffed dead cells. You need to buff-away those outer layers, regularly.

A rough washcloth is a child's introduction to *thinning*. Other thinning tools include sponges, like the loofah, brushes, and rough towels for vigorous buffing and abrasive substances such as grains and scrubs (almond meal or pumice in a rinseable base). The process of shaving facial or body hair inadvertently thins, while it removes hair.

Always protect your face from sunlight after thinning.

Masks and facials are refreshing but unnecessary. Results are most-often temporary. Don't use them if your skin is delicate and given to broken capillaries (tiny red spiderwebs just under the skin). Mint masks are particularly harmful, as is any mask, freshener or after-shave that causes a prolonged cooling or tingling sensation. These contain aromatics that can cause blood vessel damage. Avoid them.

Don't touch your skin roughly. A cosmetologist once joked that she could identify a T-1 by the quick, rough manner in which she stripped makeup from her face. No other Type is so careless with delicate skin. You help make your own wrinkles.

Don't touch your skin casually. Pushing or tugging one's earlobes, eyebrow or lower lip would seem a strange pastime, but such mannerisms are common. You may place cheek on fist, forehead on palm, or chin in hands. Ask a friend to mention every time you touch your face. Good habits can replace bad ones, and this bad habit encourages dirt, infection and wrinkles. It's worth replacing.

Satisfy skin needs. All the skin on your body needs to be clean, smooth and buffed with its moisture sealed in and its acid-mantle (the skin's surface) kept at 4.5 pH. Further, it needs freedom from dryness, abrasion, dampness, heat, cold and exposure to sunlight. Two valuable products which can ease your skin are talcum and petroleum jelly.

Talcum, cornstarch or baby powder perform beautifully as an after-bath smoother, deodorizer, sweat-absorber in shoes and underclothes, cooler of summer-hot sheets, face powder and even as an eyelash thickener before mascara.

Petroleum jelly rehabilitates dry hands and feet, softens cuticles, adds gleam to lips (put in a tiny pot with some red food coloring if you like—inexpensive lip gloss), protects nipples and thighs from abrasion when jogging, lubricates the posts on pierced earrings, removes eye makeup, conditions eyelashes, tames eyebrows and adds gleam to eyelids.

Your Skin Works Hard. Your nearly 3,000 square inches of skin is the fastest-aging organ in your body and in the most vulnerable location. No other organ is exposed. Skin helps control your temperature, warns of interior or exterior trouble, keeps infections out and our innards in, and even assists in voiding body wastes. You can't do without it, so give it every chance to be smooth, moist, glowing—a beauty asset!

Hands and feet are skin areas which require specific attention. They're discussed next.

## 19

Your Hands and Feet

Feet hide during most of the year, but hands are constantly on view. They advertise your health, age, and also your emotional state: peace, tension, enthusiasm, boredom or determination. Check your hands to see what message they are sending. You may be surprised.

The skin on hands is most threatened of all skin areas. Its enemies include soap, detergent, cleansers, sanitizers, furniture polish, paint, paint removers and thinners, cuticle remover, fruit and vegetble juices, sun, sweat, heat and cold. You can think of others.

Whenever you wash your hands, push back the cuticles with a towel. Next, *moisturize* to retain the liquid left on the skin and also prevent dryness and chapping.

Protect your hands before hand-damaging jobs by removing your rings and slipping hands into thin disposable plastic gloves or into clean cotton gloves which fit into larger rubber ones. You need insulation between your hands and negative environments. The heat and perspiration that often collects inside gloves is particularly irritating; so limit your wearing time to less than an hour.

Before working on machinery, digging in the yard, or beginning other dirty jobs where gloves are insufficient or impractical, slather your hands with a rich handcream and rake your nails across a bar of soap. This makes cleanup quicker and kinder to hands and nails.

Hands cut and bruise easily. Therefore, look before reaching into pockets, handbags and overfull drawers. Be especially careful when handling paper.

If your hands are stained, bleach them with the cut side of a lemon. It's mild.

For temporary relief of dark "liver" spots on the backs of hands try Frances Denney's *Fade-Away*® or a similar product. With twice-a-day application you should see results in just a few days, have ten-years-younger hands in three to six weeks. It's expensive, and when you stop the applications the spots will return. Discontinue using this or any product if itching or redness occurs.

Dermatologists use cryo-surgery to permanently remove dark spots. This is freezing each one with liquid nitrogen. You'll have scabbed hands for a time and suffer some discomfort, but your worst spots will be gone. After the areas have healed, additional ones can be removed if you wish. Protect those hands. Sunlight will manufacture new brownspots if you don't.

— NAILS —

Fingernails are designed to protect sensitive nerve endings, not to pry, scrape or cut. Fingerpads are designed for grasping items and have adapted well to typing and playing the piano.

Protect your nails by substituting a tool in place of a finger nail. Use a pencil or pen for dialing the telephone, a knife for opening mail and packages, and a screwdriver and small pliers for maintenance. Have these helpers in kitchen, shop, car and office. Tuck an emeryboard into every available drawer, for filing away roughness the moment you feel it will save both nails and clothing.

For nail care, assemble: cotton-tipped swabs, orange sticks, cotton balls, emery boards, a Hindostone (the fine, narrow whetstone available at beauty supply houses), petroleum jelly, cuticle remover, and diagonal pointed full-jaw nail nippers. Those wearing polish will also need: oily polish remover (choose one without acetone), tissue, base coat, polish, topcoat, and an instant-dry product (optional). Arrange your nail supplies in a tray, box or container which forms a portable manicuring kit.

To Remove Old Polish:

1. Soak two cotton balls in polish remover. Squeeze out excess remover and place one ball on each of two adjoining fingernails. Leave for a moment.

2. Wipe polish from one nail, turn cotton ball and place it on your next unstripped nail. Repeat until nails are clear of polish. Refresh balls with remover or replace them as needed. *Polish remover is bad for nails; so limit your use to once a week, please.*

3. Soak nails for five minutes in warm, soapy water. Wash away soil and remover. If you don't plan to continue your nail care until tomorrow, cream your hands with petroleum jelly, slip them into gloves and wish them a beautifying night. Or, if there's still day left, rub a pH-balanced moisturizer into hands, arms, elbows.

You fellows may not have polish to remove, but the soaking, scrubbing and moisturizing will do wonders for hands that show signs of mistreatment. The next steps are definitely unisex.

1. When nails are soft from bathing or soaking, trim them to desired length with nail clippers or scissors. Let them dry thoroughly before the next step.

2. Using the rough side of an emery board and filing in only one direction (side to center), file across your nail tip with board slanted 45 degrees toward your nailpad. Never file the sides of the nail. You need the sides to support the tip. Turn the emery board over to its finer side and smooth any rough edges. Men contour nails to the shape of their fingertips, women to somewhat-flattened ovals. No blunt-cuts nor stilettos!

3. Dip the tapered end of your Hindostone into cuticle remover or warm water and use it as a pencil eraser to gently nudge-back and grind-away your cuticle. Old polish and stains will also come away with gentle abrasion. Now dip your Hindostone in water and use the tapered end to refile the underside edge of your nailtip, and finally the nail's surface. They must be smooth.

4. Snip any hangnails with the diagonal nail nippers. Trim away any next-to-nail calluses. No major surgery, please.

5. Wash your hands. Push back your cuticles as you dry them.

6. Buffing the nails is optional. A high shine can be obtained with nail-buffing kits, but it's not recommended for those with delicate nails or those wishing to top their shine with polish. Polish won't always adhere.

7. Cream hands, arms, and elbows.

Nail polish is also unisex, for men often like a clear glaze finish to protect their nails. But women have the latitude. Their choice of color in nail polish is staggering.

T-1s choose clear or cream enamel in skintone or reds. T-2s look for clear, cream, and pearlized polish in skintones and reds. T-3s wear clear, cream, and metallic polishes in skintones, reds, and their more exotic colors. T-4s select clear, cream, pearl, or frost enamels in skintone, silver, or reds. But everyone be warned, frost and pearlized polish is harder on the nails than cream and clear. Always undercoat.

Beautiful hands and fingers are best displayed with bright polish and interesting rings and bracelets. Less attractive hands and fingers are best disguised with clear or skin-tone polishes and a limited amount of simple jewelry.

Nail polish forms a protective coating on nails and lessens the chance of breaking, splitting and peeling. It thus earns itself a place on most women's "important to do" list whether they seek glamour or not.

Apply polish professionally.

1. Dip a cotton-tipped swab in polish remover and carefully clean each fingernail of possible oil. Wash your hands and dry them—pushing back all cuticles. Let nails dry thoroughly before polishing.

2. Apply a thin *base coat* in four motions: down the center of the nails from base to tip, a stroke on either side and a bit under the tip to reduce chipping. One dip of your brush should do one nail. Begin with the brush in your most awkward hand. Paint your thumbnail first, your little finger's nail next, and then ring finger to pointer. Switch hands and repeat.

3. Roll *polish* between your palms. Don't shake it or stir the polish with its brush. Apply your favorite color in the same manner you did the base. If you should accidentally flood the nail, pick up excess polish with the point of an orange stick run around the cuticle. Wipe the orange stick on a tissue. Never apply color directly to your nails. You need a base coat to help polish adhere and to protect your nails from staining.

4. Apply a second coat of color. Let this coat dry for fifteen minutes.

5. Top with a coat of clear sealer to protect nails and prevent your polish from chipping. Let dry for twenty minutes before you use your hands normally. A book or magazine nearby encourages carefulness. Or wait one minute before spraying or coating your wet polish with a quick-dry product. Keep chores light and hands out of water for at least two hours. Ban hot baths or heavy housework for at least twelve hours. Polish needs time to thoroughly harden.

6. Every day or two add a coat of polish and sealer (if chips are present), or sealer alone. Always make certain your nails are oil-free before you add another coat. Your manicure should last seven-ten days.

Persistent nail problems are often the first sign of interior trouble. Doublecheck your diet, fresh air and exercise, then see a doctor or dermatologist if trouble persists. Gelatine has not proven effective in controlled medical tests. It's not the secret to stronger nails.

Nails won't grow? Illness and emotional upsets affect the health of your nails, and rates of growth vary. You can count on a growth of 1/4 inch a month during normal times, if you're average. Pregnancy speeds up the growth rate to double, and childbirth slows it way down.

False fingernails might be a solution to nibbled or broken nails. You can glue on plastic nails or a professional can build sculptured nails on top of your own. But since nails grow, a noticeable gap will form between your cuticle and the manufactured nail. This gap must be filled every 2 weeks—a cost in time and money. The fakes often teach their owners to protect their hands, to gesture more gracefully, and actually to grow longer nails. But, conversely, they're potentially harmful and can't be adopted permanently.

Discolored nails? Gently bleach nails with white iodine (available at your druggist). One drop massaged into each nail then rinsed off should solve your problem. You can prevent discoloration by using a basecoat under dark or bright polishes and choosing a polish-remover free of acetone.

Splitting nails? Don't try to cut-off the offending portion. Reattach it with a nail mending or patching kit according to package directions. Use after removing your old polish and before adding new. Optionally, if you're feeling wealthy, consider having your nails "wrapped" by a professional manicurist. Wrapping each nailtip prevents splitting and breakage.

Finally, use lots of petroleum jelly, cuticle cream or moisturizer on your hands and cuticles. They'll thrive on it.

— FEET —

Look at your feet. Are they smooth, soft and well-proportioned? Or are they less-than-perfect in conformation, or callused and rough? If the former is the case, wear distinctive sandals, go barefoot at the least provocation, display them. If the latter is the case, don't subject others to the sight of your feet. Cover them up. If your feet fall in-between and are barely adequate, choose skintone sandals in the summer.

You can't change too-long or too-short toes, but you can care for your feet and make them smooth and neat.

To improve your feet:

Choose stockings and shoes 1/2 inch longer than your feet.

Select shoes that fit correctly. Ninety-five percent of the 500 possible foot ailments come from incorrect fit.

Change socks or stockings daily.

Remove fashion boots at least once during the day. Wriggle your toes and massage your feet to increase circulation.

Avoid wearing rubber boots over long periods of time. Feet can't breathe in them.

Change your shoes often.

Four-inch and higher heels are harmful for those with short feet. They look ill-proportioned, too.

Walk barefoot around your house or apartment, daily. Also walk barefoot in the sand whenever you can.

If you have corns or thick calluses, visit a podiatrist. He'll start you off on a personal footcare plan.

Normal footcare, performed daily, includes: bathing for cleanliness, pumicing for callus removal, creaming for retaining moisture and powder for protection.

Every third week set aside time for a pedicure.

Pedicuring.

1. Remove old polish as you did your nail polish.

2. Soak feet in warm, sudsy water or water with a foot-soak preparation added, for at least fifteen minutes. Scrub away soil with a washcloth or brush. Wear-down your calluses with a wet pumice stone or a "hard skin reducer" (available in dime and drug stores). Clean under your nailtips with a sudsy cotton-wrapped swab.

3. Dry feet, pushing back the cuticles.

4. Clip your toenails, just shorter than your toes, and leave the corners square to discourage ingrown nails.

5. Smooth nailtips with an emeryboard, but don't round the corners.

6. Massage cuticle remover all around your cuticles. Gently push back cuticles with a wet Hindostone. Smooth all nail surfaces and tips.

7. Scrub your toes, washing away cuticle remover and dead skin. Dry thoroughly.

8. Massage petroleum jelly or rich cream into legs and feet. Slip socks on your feet and wear them overnight if you can. You'll love the way your feet feel in the morning.

To Polish Toenails:

1. Dip a cotton-tipped swab into polish remover and clean nail surfaces of oil. Rinse toes. Dry thoroughly, pushing back cuticles.

2. Twist a tissue and weave it between the toes of each foot. This makes polish application easier and neater.

3. Apply a base coat, two coats of enamel and one clear topcoat. Make certain each coat is dry before you apply the next. Note: red toenails add a delightfully feminine accent peeping from strappy shoes. Use one of your reds. It needn't match your fingernail polish.

4. Relax, legs elevated, until polish dries.

\# \# \# \# \#

The next chapter deals with your hair. Did you know that hairstyles, too, can be divided into 4 Types? They can and will be on the next pages.

20

Your Hair

The hair on your head has no practical value. It's no longer needed as insulation from heat or cold nor to warn of a low cave entrance. But oh, the psychological comfort! And hair can work wizardry in transforming the ordinary face and head into the fabulous. The merest hint of hair's loss lends trauma.

What are the needs of your hair? How can you protect it, groom it, and style it to give yourself the most pleasure? Read on.

Hair is dead protein with a pH of 4.5 to 5.5. At proper pH it has optimum elasticity, strength and luster; so choose hair products that share this same pH range.

You can count on your hair growing approximately one-half inch a month. If you shaved shoulder-length hair to star in a science-fiction television thriller, you'd wait two years for it to grow back to its original length. Don't be surprised if you can't grow long, long hair. Women's hair rarely grows longer than three feet.

Expect more rapid growth in summer and when you're pregnant, a corresponding loss of hair in fall and after childbirth.

Of the 100,000 hair follicles on an average head, 85 percent will contain growing hair. The balance will be dormant. Fortunately, the growing period lasts two to six years and the dormant stage averages only three months. Plus, your follicles are generally kind enough to stagger their vacations.

Like your skin, hair follicles are highly sensitive to diet and emotional disturbances.

Hair loss caused by anemia, low thyroid function, and estrogen deficiency is reversible when the problem is corrected. If you have weak-follicles, they were inherited from your parents. Nothing can be done to increase numbers and quality of hair . . . no cure, yet, for male-patterned baldness. Sorry. But a loss of 100 to 150 hairs a day is normal for everyone.

Beautiful hair is clean, free, bouncy, and natural. It's also delicate as cobwebs of silk. Eat well for your hair's sake. And protect your hair from heat, cold, sun, wind, perspiration, chlorine, saltwater, dirt, tangling, teasing, alkaline products, brush curlers, enthusiastic brushing, excessive coloring, curling or straightening, crash diets, rubber bands, ponytails, and tight wigs and caps.

— SHAMPOOING —

Shampoo your hair when it's dirty, limp, or oily—every day if you like. Use a pair of shampoos which test pH 4.5 and alternate them every few days. Both can be diluted by half with water. If you suds your head daily, try the mild, for-dry-hair shampoos and apply only *once*. Don't strip away natural oils with strong shampoos and excessive lathering.

Going from dingy to shining hair:

1. Comb or lightly brush dirt, hairspray and tangles from your hair. Make certain the teeth of your comb and bristles of your brush aren't sharp. If they hurt your fingers, they'll hurt your hair.

2. Wet your hair with a gentle stream of lukewarm water, never hot.

3. Pour a small amount of *shampoo* into your palm, rub your hands together, then stroke them the length of your hair. Work up a suds while keeping hairshafts as straight as possible. Massage shampoo into your scalp with the pads of your fingers. Work gently but quickly. Shampoo is necessary, but it's not completely kind.

4. Rinse out the shampoo again, again, and again.

5. Pour a small amount of pH balanced *conditioner* into your palm. Stroke it repeatedly the length of your hair, but avoid your scalp. Separate the strands of hair, finger-combing. Leave conditioner on as long as directions indicate. (Wash your comb and brush while you wait). Blacks can't afford to miss this step since their hair is usually brittle and prone to break. Conditioning reduces tangling and static, restores shine and manageability.

6. Rinse completely. When you've finished rinsing, rinse some more—this time with cool water. Make it as cold as you can stand, for low temperatures firm the hairshaft. If your wet hair looks dull, you haven't rinsed enough.

7. Blot the moisture from your hair with an absorbent towel. Don't rub. Take a second towel and make a turban to wear while your hair goes from wet to damp. Unwrap.

8. Don't ever brush wet hair—it breaks too easily. But you can carefully run a wide-toothed comb through damp locks. If you find tangles, gently work them out from the ends up, not from the scalp down.

9. Afros should be styled when wet or damp. Use tortoiseshell, rubber or plastic combs with your fluffy style. Metal combs can damage hair.

10. Dry your hair as gently and slowly as possible. Air drying would be a first choice provided you have the style and time that allows it. A second choice would be drying under a heatlamp. Many bathrooms have them in the ceiling vent with blower and light.

11. Last choices include in descending order and with heat control turned low: blow dryers, bonnet dryers, and heated rollers. Never dry your hair bone-dry with heat. Let room-temperature air cool your hair as it draws off the last bit of moisture.

When using a blowdryer, hold it six to ten inches away from your hair and keep it moving. A motionless dryer can damage both scalp and hair. For a sleek look, brush and blow in the direction your hair falls. For a full, bouncy look, brush and blow in the opposite direction. Set your dryer on warm for styling and on cool to lock in the finished shape. Cool air makes your set last longer.

Watch how your stylist operates with brush and blower. Ask questions. With practice you can duplicate professional results at home. Also note the brands and types of products used and try similar products at home. Experiment with products and techniques until you have an unbeatable hair-care combination.

If you use hairspray to control flyaway wisps, hold it at least twelve inches away from your hair. Any closer and it saturates your hair and scalp. A fine mist is optimum. Close your eyes when you spray to keep from irritating them. And, for the hair's sake, comb hairspray out each bedtime.

— HAIR DIFFERENCES —

Those with naturally bouncy, sleek hair may wish to eliminate some or all of the recommended conditioning. Those with dry, damaged hair may wish to add a monthly deep-conditioning treatment to their routine. Look for pH balanced products that are applied warm or that are applied, then wrapped with a hot towel for a period of time.

Dandruff flakes on the navy flannel indicate that you need a specialized shampoo. Look for those containing any of the following: selenium, zinc, tar, sulfur or salicylic acid. Sulfur is said to be quite helpful. Select two good dandruff-removing shampoos with differing ingredients and alternate between them. But, since dandruff shampoos are naturally drying, use a regular shampoo occasionally. Careful conditioning with a rinse-out type conditioner can also block hair dryness. If after three weeks of home treatment you still have dandruff, see your dermatologist.

Split-ends don't just lie there. They travel up the shaft toward the scalp. A good conditioner will help them be less noticeable, but only two things will stop their motion: trimming off the splits or singeing. Both processes should be done by a professional. If your hair tends to split, use electric rollers and curling irons sparingly, and shampoo less often and more gently.

Baby-fine hair needs frequent shampooing. Avoid *cream* rinses and conditioners. Choose body-building conditioners, instead. A blunt cut works particularly well. A body wave can lend manageability and apparent thickening. It won't last much more than two months, however, and the process shouldn't be repeated in less than four months.

Fine, limp, virgin hair can have increased body for most of the year with treatments of neutral henna. (Find it in the beauty supply house.) This doesn't change your hair's color, only its thickness. If overused, henna is drying, so limit it as you do permanents. Never use henna on permanented, straightened or colored hair. And purchase the neutral, not the colors!

Thin, spare hair calls for very gentle handling and a short, blunt-cut style. Avoid body waves and henna unless hair is in excellent condition. Try bangs or hairpieces. Also try Jhirmack's *Uphold*, a wave set gelee. Rub a pencil eraser amount of this pink jell between your finger tips before stroking through untangled clean, dry hair. Let dry. Comb. Style. It adds body and helps retain the styling.

Coarse hair goes wiry if cut too short, and wild if cut too long. Keep it chin to shoulder length. Use cream rinses and conditioners to soften it and big rollers to give direction.

Very curly hair loves a short, layered cut. Choose a wash-and-wear style and let it curl.

Thick hair should be trimmed frequently and kept fairly short. Never let it be thinned.

Overworked, dry lifeless hair needs trimming into a wash-and-wear style, lots of moisturizing conditioners and avoidance of chemicals such as coloring, permanents, straightening and heat from dryers, curling irons and heated rollers. If you want to escape baldness, let all processed hair grow out. Then protect your new hair.

Oily hair must be shampooed often. Consider ending your shampoos with a rinse solution made up of juice from a lemon squeezed into one cup of lukewarm water. Leave it on your hair for five minutes. Rinse with cool water. Avoid hot dryers. A neutral henna treatment is a possibility if your hair is "virgin."

Flyaway Hair stays in place with a light misting of water—use a spray-top bottle. Substitute a rubber comb for your plastic one to keep down static electricity.

Cowlicks part your hair without permission. Best solution is to comb as *they* like. A body permanent will turn them around temporarily but not permanently.

— PROFILE IRREGULARITIES —

Hair is the best possible makeup to contour, soften, disguise, and display your features; and it also balances body proportions. Those who are:

Tall look best in medium-to-long hair, styled with some bulk. Those with larger features and regal bearing also enjoy sleek, controlled styles.

Short require neat, short hair and "up" styles.

Overweight need hairstyles to balance their silhouette. Keep hair full and rounded, but off the shoulders.

Long, thin necked are most attractive with hair brushing the sides of their necks.

Short necked lengthen apparent neck with short and upswept hair.

Broad shouldered with a thick neck need soft, diagonal waves and a full hairdo with diagonal lines.

Lacking in chin add hair fullness at the crown.

Over-supplied with chin keep curls at the chinline, sleekness at the crown.

Receding or bulging in forehead hide under bangs and dress nape hair close to the head.

Large nosed arrange fullness around the face with flatness at the back of the head. Or, they may sleek the hair back into a classic chignon. An important nose can be a beauty signature.

Puffy eyed forget bangs and brush hair up and away from the face.

— FACIAL SHAPES —

If you don't recognize your face shape when hearing geometric terms, pull out your "facial photo." Cover it with tracing paper and trace the outline of your face. Remove your portrait and you'll see something on the tracing that is similar to an oval, circle, square, rectangle, diamond, triangle or heart. To discover the shape of your face you may need to eliminate what it isn't. Does that work any better?

The ideal facial shape is oval, and hair can give the illusion that every face is an oval. Here's the system.

The oval face is lucky. It can wear most hairstyles.

The round face needs fullness at chin and crown, narrowness at cheekbone. Hair may cover the sides of the face.

The square face looks best in asymmetric styles which soften the corners.

The long face avoids a center-part, needs volume on the sides to make a full, rounded impression.

The diamond face chooses bangs plus fullness at chin level to widen narrow areas.

The triangular face has a narrow forehead and wide jaw. This face is enhanced with horizontal bangs to widen above the eyes and fullness on the cheeks.

The heart-shaped face has width through the forehead that tapers to a pointed chin. Best balance is with full hair below the temples.

— MATCHING YOUR TYPE —

Early in this book relationships between your personality, bone structure, and coloring were established. You identified your Type and learned how to choose clothing which complimented you. Now, choose a hairstyle that repeats the statement you and your apparel are making.

Type One hair is generally smooth and shiny with little curl, but amount of curl varies. You can be a T-1 and have tight curls.

Men of this Type choose well-cut, young hairstyles. Controlled with a light misting of hairspray or blow-dry touseled, it looks clean, crisp and healthy—like the fellow-next-door's hair should look.

Type One women are prettiest in rounded, smooth, fluffy, curly, wavy, or flippy styles like Orphan Annie, the Dutch Boy, a twenties bob, a curly cap, boy-cuts, shoulder-length swing, long and curly, pageboy, short and brushed up—all young and perky.

Hairtrimming for T-1 includes bows, butterflies, flowers, barrettes, bright combs, headbands, scarves as headbands, ribbons and yarn.

Type Two hair is often fine as gossamer. It needs gentle handling and romantic styling.

T-2 males look like nobility. They choose slightly longer hair, soft waves, and even moustaches and "period" beards add to their specialness.

The women are meltingly feminine in shoulder-length hair with "S" curves, waves, curls, tendrils beside the face, soft French twists, loose chignons, side twists, soft rolls and silhouettes forming ovals.

Hair trims include delicate flowers and combs, velvet ribbons, silken cords and veiling.

Type Three hair is usually thick and wiry. Always vibrant, it can be tamed into a

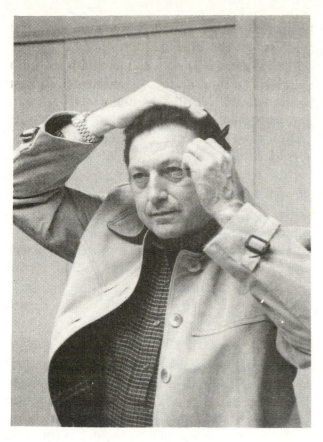

T-3 grooming hair

smooth shape or allowed a limited freedom to explode.

Males of the harmony wear a wide variety of casual hairstyles from the smooth-top of T-3s Yul Brenner and Telly Savalas to tousled manes.

T-3 women exude earthiness or excitement in angular shapes with diagonal lines. Curly Afro, lion's mane, Grecian, frenzy, Indian braids, crimped twists, and simple diagonally-parted flip, chin-length bob, short brush-up and no-part shoulder length are some of their choices.

Hair trimmings include exotic or tortoiseshell combs, leather clamps or thongs, feathers, metallic chains or braids, chopsticks, shells, and flashes of metal.

Type Four hair is classically smooth and straight, but all T-4s don't have classic hair.

T-4 men need expert and frequent cutting, for neither stray hair nor overdue haircut is acceptable with their contrast drawing the spotlight. Aim for sculptured neatness.

T-4 women frame their faces with sleek effects like a smooth chignon, roll or twist; a shiny cap; a center-parted flip with horizontal motion, a Cleopatra bob. They choose either classic simplicity or a strikingly contemporary form.

Hair trimmings are a diamond tiara or nothing.

— OCCASION —

One becoming hairdo can be worn at all hours and for all occasions, as you men have certainly proven. And those with difficult or damaged hair should locate their one style and not change it. But you can decide if adopting a second, more important, hairstyle for festive occasions is worth considering.

Whether you need one becoming hairstyle or two, once again bring out facial photos and tracing paper.

Slip tracing paper over your full-face photo, trace your features and hairline, then sketch the hairdos you've considered while reading this chapter. Try several with more paper. You'll soon judge whether A is better than C. Now, sketch the best styles on a tracing covering your profile photo. Do your best styles pass the test? Great. You may have designed your perfect hairstyle or two. If they require the same length and shape of hair, you'll be able to use them interchangeably.

Unless you shun beaches, lakes, and pools, you'll need to plan for soaking wet hair in public. Hats, scarves, wigs, and sleekly-combed hair are obvious choices. Try them and select the most becoming. Be ready for the unexpected.

You've finished the do-it-yourself portion of this subject. Now you need professional assistance.

— HAIRCUTS —

The most ideal style for your hair is one that considers fineness/coarseness, thinness/thickness, straightness/curliness, and condition while complementing your facial shape, head and body size, and Type. It should look

119

good wet as well as dry. You may have predetermined the style you want, but you definitely require the services of a superior hair cutter.

How do you find this paragon? Look at your friends, acquaintances and total strangers. When you see someone with a great cut, ask who did it. People are flattered to be asked. If his/her hair is like yours, ask for a name to give the stylist. The more expensive salons tend to have the better stylists, but secure a hair cutting genius or fine barber wherever you find one. Don't skimp on the cost of a haircut. Wash and dry it yourself if you need to economize.

Meet the stylist in your street clothes before your hair has been wet. Your body shape and lifestyle are a part of the total look to be developed.

Ask for a trim at first to see if work is precise and if the two of you are on the same wave length. Explain your hair's peculiarities, your skill in handling your hair, what you like and dislike, how you'd like to look. Show pictures and clippings of styles you've been considering and perhaps your sketches. Discuss the direction you'll take at the next appointment.

Watch what is done and ask how to care for your hair at home. If you can't manage your hair, you're handicapped in this time of stepped-up activity and travel.

Plan on having your hair cut or trimmed every four to six weeks whether it's short-short or you're sitting on it. Hair needs regular trimming for health. Keep an eye on fashion trends and modify yours when hairstyles go smaller or larger. Or if you find the perfect style, you can keep it as a signature for a lifetime.

— PERMANENTS —

Permanents curl straight hair and give body to fine or thin hair. They help your hair to turn the direction you and your stylist wish it to go. On short cuts, permanents allow you to towel-try your curls and go—frizz perhaps but no blowing, no work. They help sets stay in. For a time you are a curly head or at least the possessor of a fatter head of hair.

Unfortunately hair grows, moving the curls away from your scalp at the rate of 6 inches a year, leaving hair that doesn't curl. Permanents damage the hairshaft and the damage remains until the permanent grows out. It's dangerous to reperm damaged hair or bleach it or color it. Retreating hair is best not done, but if you must, put your hair in the hands of an expert or you may find your hair in your hands. You'll have awkward between-permanent periods and unless you know your operator, you run the risk of frizzies.

Recent tests have proven that a person who is pH-balanced has far better success with permanents; so check your pH just before being permanented. A little Nitrazine paper on your tongue will indicate if you are as well-balanced as your shampoo. If needed, correct your pH to 5.5 or 6.0 with a glass of orange juice or a snack of apple before you leave for your appointment.

Virgin hair, given proper care and styling, is lovelier, but permanents are an option. Caution: they should never be used when you color your hair . . . both processes damage hair and the combination can be disastrous.

— HAIR COLOR —

Hair coloring is now a major industry which whispers from TV screen, magazine and newspaper pages, "Changing your hair color will improve your life." Don't believe it. Changing your hair color will cost you repeated investments of time and money. It leaves hair dry and lifeless. Poorly chosen haircolors detract from the face, and even well-chosen haircolors are changed by time, sunlight, chlorine and shampooing to metallic tones you don't bargain for. The contrast between dyed hair and new growth? Ugly.

But don't blondes have more fun? Not necessarily. Confidence in oneself lends pizazz in social relationships. Looking like yourself and loving it beats changing your appearance to match someone else's criteria. Besides, you've already learned that contrast of dark and light is more eye-catching than bright color. Why eliminate the only contrast you have? Those who lighten mid-range hair lose contrast and trade their individuality for paperdoll sameness.

But what about grey hair? It's kind and, if well-groomed, beautiful. As you age not only does your hair show strands of white but your skin and eyes gently fade. They don't change hue—become more yellow or red—they lose intensity and value. Dyeing hair to its former color is unkind to skin and eyes, and going blonde ages one. The natural lightening of your hair will keep pace with skin and eyes—leaving you balanced. Styling and caring for your gray, partially gray or white hair will leave you beautiful.

The four types gray differently. Type Fours gain a beautiful mane after a striking salt and pepper era. T-3s' hair turns to incomparable tweed. The ashen locks of T-2 become more ashen . . . lighter and softer. Type One journeys from color to white over various roads, depending upon ancestry.

White or almost-white hair sometimes yellows—a less than attractive change caused by smog or fumes. For these individuals a toner can cut the yellow. Revlon's Tone-up #52, Artic White, a white white, used sparingly, is one to try.

And don't worry. The "Becoming Colors" which formerly flattered remain flattering throughout all natural hair-face changes—even to the whitest of hair.

Hair is an attractive frame for the subject of the next chapter, your face.

21

Your Face

A mirror image greets you each time you shave, apply makeup, wash hands, brush teeth, or comb your hair. But do you actually *see* the face you wear? Should you?

Recognition of facial symmetry and irregularity is fully as important as isolating your body's strong and weak points. You use clothing to give an illusion of perfection. Makeup and facial hair can, likewise, maximize facial assets and minimize its handicaps.

Understanding your countenance is more important than owning the rare face with perfect features. And that understanding of your face will be yours, shortly.

You'll need a pencil, ruler, your front-view facial photo, tracing paper and masking tape. Or in place of the tape and tracing paper, you can duplicate your facial photo on a copy machine. The image won't be completely clear, but it will be adequate. The chart you make will resemble the illustration on page 123.

— SPOTTING IRREGULARITIES —

1. Place a sheet of tracing paper over your front view photo and secure it with tape, so it can't slide—if you've opted not to copy your photo.

2. Draw a dotted horizontal line across your tracing at the level of your center-front hairline.

3. Draw a second dotted horizontal at the level of the bottom inside edge of your eyebrows.

4. Draw a third dotted horizontal at the bottom of your nose.

5. Draw a fourth dotted horizontal at the bottom of your lower lip.

6. Draw a fifth dotted horizontal at the bottom of your chin.

7. Measure the actual distances between each pair of horizontal dotted lines and record them in the left margin.

8. Draw dotted vertical lines at the inside and outside of each eye, extending from the top to the bottom of your tracing or sheet.

9. Measure the distance between your eyes and the width of your eye. Record in the right margin with those measurements labeled.

10. Draw a pair of dotted diagonal lines from the sides of your nostrils past the outside edge of your eyes, extending into your hair.

11. Draw dotted vertical lines from the center of each nostril to the bottom of your lower lip.

12. Draw a short dotted vertical line on the upper lip, midway between the existing vertical lines.

13. Place dots at the outside corners of your mouth, slightly higher than the actual corners.

14. Measure the width of your face and record it in the bottom margin. Label it "width."

15. Measure the length of your face and record it, labeled, in the bottom margin.

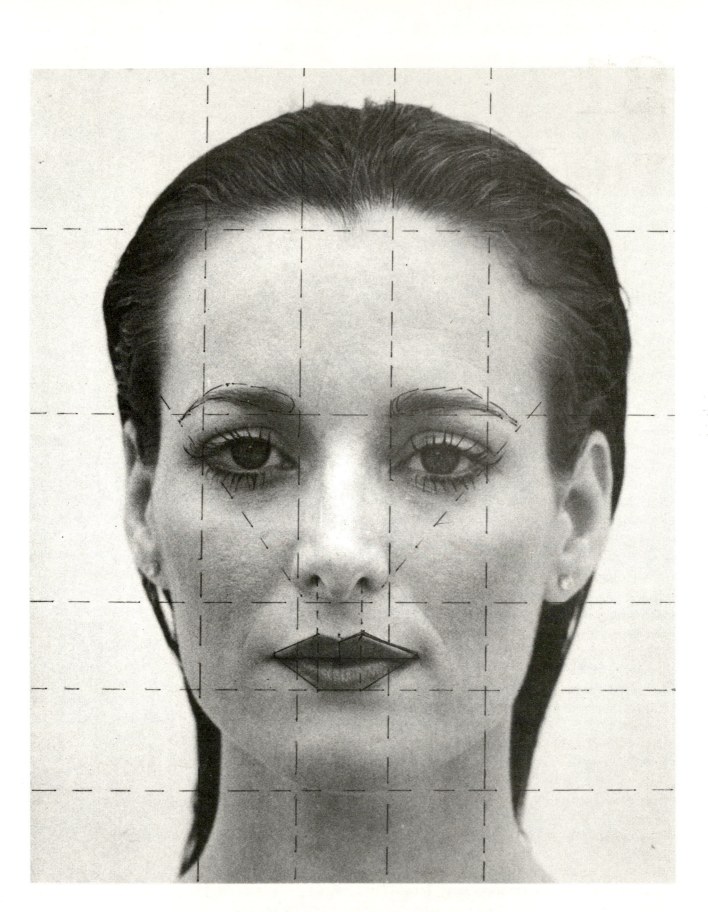

Facial Chart of a T-1 with T-3 bones and T-4 skin

123

— EVALUATING RESULTS —

The four horizontal lines at hairline, eyebrow, nose and chin ideally divide the face into three equal parts. If your face is evenly divided, rejoice. If you have one section that's longer than the others, write LONG in the left margin. If shorter, write SHORT. If all three are different measurements, write LONG on the longest and SHORT on the shortest.

Don't worry if your facial divisions are unequal. You've lots of company.

Now check the measurements between nose/bottom lip and bottom lip/chin. Ideally they're equal. If yours aren't, write LONG or SHORT in the left margin.

The width between your eyes and the width of your eye is ideally equal. If your eyes are wider than the space between write CLOSE-SET EYES in the left margin. If the area between your eyes is wider than your eye, write WIDE-SET eyes.

Divide the width of your face by its length. The perfect oval would be .75, a ratio of three to four. Write your ratio by the dimensions and add IDEAL, SLIGHTLY BROAD or VERY NARROW, whatever is indicated.

— MAKING A FACIAL CHART —

Brows: Eyebrows are tremendously important to your face for they're viewed as indicators of both intelligence and grooming. Further, they're said to control 25 percent of your facial expression. No wonder they can enhance or destroy impact.

The starting point for normal brows is indicated by the vertical lines you've drawn at the inside edges of your eyes. If you have *wide-set eyes*, your brows should start inside that line, *the width of your eye apart*. If your eyes are *close-set*, start your brows outside that line, *the width of the eye apart*. The beginning of the brow is rounded, not square-cut. Place curved lines where your brows should begin.

The diagonal lines from the sides of your nostrils past the outside edge of your eyes sig-nal the end of the brow. Brows never stop abruptly but fade-out so gradually you don't notice. Place a dot where your brow should end.

The highest point in the arch of the brow is normally directly above the outside of the iris. For those with *wide-set* eyes, the arch can start sooner and peak above the inner edge of the pupil. For those with *close-set* eyes, the outer edge of the eye is most becoming as a high point to the arch. Place a dot on or slightly above the upper curve of your brow-line to indicate the high point of the arch.

Draw the curve of your upper brow, connecting the center curve with the dots. You should have a long, bent angle with curved, not straight, sides. Now draw the underbrow. When completed, you have a long, bent triangle.

Play with various brow thicknesses until you have a design that becomes your face, but retain your upper brow line. Drawing narrower brows means increasing the distance between eye and brow by eliminating a portion of the *underneath* hairs. Brows are only plucked from the undercurve—never from the upper. Eyebrow pencil can add any brows you lack.

If your brows are distinctive, a la Margo Hemingway, and you wish to retain their character, do so. Forget the sketched brow. Violating rules is fine if you know them first and are willing to take the risk.

Postpone the decision about your brows, if you wish, or use an eyebrow pencil to draw the perfect brow on your face. See if you like your new brow's shape better than you do your familiar one. You can always scrub it off—no harm done.

— GROOMING BROWS —

Normal eyebrows and lashes grow for ten weeks then rest for nine months, but they'll seem to be sprouting daily. Plan to pluck strays at least weekly at a time other than when you apply makeup. The equipment you'll need for brow grooming includes: an icecube, cotton balls, alcohol, a pair of *slant-nosed* tweezers, antiseptic cream or petroleum jelly, a mirror and good light. A magnifying mirror is especially helpful.

1. Wipe the tweezer tips in alcohol-soaked cotton.

2. Cleanse your brow area the same way.

3. Chill the underbrow or the area between brows with the icecube.

4. Stretch the brow taut with your opposite hand while grasping each individual hair. Pluck in the direction hair grows.

5. When you reshape your brows, remove only one hair deep, beginning at the center and working outward. Repeat for other brow. Evaluate. Brows should look natural and beautiful. Take another line of hairs only if you're certain you need less brow. Evaluate. Live with these narrower brows for awhile before considering more shaping.

6. After plucking, wipe reddened areas with an alcohol-dipped cotton ball.

7. Finish with a thin coating of antiseptic cream or petroleum jelly applied to the same sites.

Lips: Draw a perfect mouth on your tracing or print by connecting the beside-mouth dots to the dotted lines where they bisect upper and lower lip edges. Keep the lines straight. They'll dip to a V in the center of your upper lip. Ideally, lips are equal in width, so slightly thicken a too-thin lip or slightly narrow a too-full one for better balance.

When your own lips are decidedly imperfect, females can disguise imperfections with makeup, males with a moustache.

A moustache is great camouflage for men with uneven mouths or excess distance between nose and lips. Sketch a moustache on your tracing if you have one or more of these problems. Try different shapes. Does a moustache improve you enough to be worth growing one?

Women can minimize nose to mouth distance by making the upper lip's V very shallow, almost non-existent. Imperfectly shaped mouths can be corrected with opaque coverup plus lipstick.

Chins: If the distance between mouth and chin is too short or long, a neatly-trimmed beard will disguise that fact. Experiment with various shapes, fellows. Women can slightly modify the width of their lips and contour their chins to gain or lose apparent chin length. You experiment, too.

Makeup has been traditionally reserved for women but is less so each year. Men have found that winter-pale can be banished with bronzers, and flaws can be disguised with contouring techniques. Men also have photo sessions or television appearances where makeup can dramatically improve their appearance.

Whatever your makeup questions, you'll find them tucked in the next chapter.

22

Your Makeup

Have you ever seen a performance of female impersonators? Your eyes and ears testify to the femininity of the talented and beautiful singers, dancers and comediennes. But late in each act the illusion is shattered by a baritone voice or an exposed male head or chest. With the deception so well-established the truth appears unbelievable.

What has that to do with you and makeup? If men can be *that* effective with makeup, wigs and clothing, there's no excuse for a woman to look less than wonderful. A man surely has a greater handicap in looking like a beautiful woman than YOU do.

What equipment and supplies are needed for professional makeup application? Nothing too exotic. You probably already own most of it.

— EQUIPMENT AND SUPPLIES —

1. *Mirror and Light*. North light is ideal, but you can substitute a good, lighted makeup mirror in a well-lit room for routine applications. Always check your face with a hand mirror and north light before important occasions. You'll find small errors you'd otherwise miss.

2. *Foundation*. Look for a water-based, translucent liquid the exact color of your face and throat or a tone that blends the several colors of your skin. Check prospective foundation colors on your neck skin at chinline. Your makeup base should be nearly invisible with a matte finish. If you tan (I don't recommend it) you'll need a second bottle, either lighter or darker, to blend with the first. By custom mixing you'll have a perfect foundation tone all year round.

If your foundation is too mask-like, carefully thin it with distilled or mineral water. As you grow older use less, not more, foundation.

3. *Makeup Sponges*. (have several) Sponges work best if small, fine and thin. If you can't find a shape you like, try cutting larger sponges to your specifications.

4. *Blemish Coverup*. This should be opaque, somewhat creamy, and the exact color of your skin or one shade lighter. It comes in tube, stick or jar.

If you have a dark birthmark, a scar or varicose veins which need hiding, look for Lydia O'Leary Covermark Corrective Cosmetics®. They're available in many shades and a wide number of products which disguise imperfections admirably.

5. *Blusher*. Choose a powder if your skin is oily or a cream version if your skin is dry. The shade should be a darker form of the red inside your lower lip. Blusher looks dark in its container, so test it on your skin before buying. Best blushes for blacks include shades of plum, bronze and amber.

6. *Eye Makeup Foundation* (optional). A matte surface on which to brush eye shadows is luxurious and helps shadow stay on. It's a necessity for those with dry and wrinkled or oily and slick lids.

7. *Eyebrow/Moustache Comb and Brush.* This double sided comb/brush is compact, inexpensive and can be found with either eyebrow or moustache tools. The brush strokes brows; the comb separates eyelashes.

8. *Eyebrow Pencil.* Your brows are tiny hairs; therefore, the pencil which imitates them needs to be sharp, so you can draw additional tiny hairs. Choose a color, or pair of colors, approximately 2-shades lighter than your hair. No black, ever!

9. *Eye-Pencil Sharpener.* Keep both the slim brow/lip and thick shadow/blush pencils pointed with an eye pencil sharpener. Buy it at the cosmetic counter.

10. *Eye Shadow Pencils or Creamy Pressed Shadows.* Eye shading is selected from your collection of skintones or neutrals. Look for muted smoky tones—no brights. Include light, medium and dark tones. Brown, charcoal, wine, olive, warm and cool grays make attractive dark shadows. Cream, light gray, lavender and taupe are equally desirable for lightness. Choose only colors you can wear.

T-4s alone can wear frosts but should use them sparingly. They're drying. Blacks look stunning in dark neutrals and should avoid pastels, blues and greens.

Try sample sizes, testers and dimestore purchases until you settle on your exact needs. Test colors on your inner arm, grouping them as you intend to wear them. Never test on your eye area. Eyes and surrounding skin are ultra sensitive to infection.

Too-bright shadows may be combined into softer tones. Use uneven amounts of complementary colors, add a drop of moisturizer and pour all into a throw-away tin. Melt the shadows, stir and pour them into a tiny container. A new color is born.

Best of all personal eye shadows is the hue exactly opposite the color-wheel from your eye color. Keep the intensity below that of your iris. Since "complements" increase apparent intensity, your eyes will look brilliant.

11. *Eyeliner* (optional). Either liquid eyeliner, which is applied with a finely pointed brush, or a pencil eyeliner should be chosen in a dark neutral shade. Use when it's fashionable. Omit when it's not.

12. *Eyelash Curler.* An eyelash curler may sound outdated, but it makes a flattering difference in your appearance. Since the rubber inserts wear out, check yours occasionally, and replace them when they become grooved—you want curled lashes, not amputated ones. Those wearing glasses will find the eyelash curler a MAJOR beauty asset.

13. *Brush Wand Mascara.* Select one of your darkest neutrals: black, brown-black, deep navy, brown or taupe. If you use a cream foundation, choose a water-based mascara. It makes lashes look thicker and is easier to remove, but must be reapplied more often. Choose a waterproof form if you wear a water-based foundation and want a truly lasting mascara. One disadvantage—it's difficult to remove.

14. *Eye Makeup Remover.* This product should remove mascara gently, without tugging at the eye-area. Look for a non-oily one. Oil-based removers are kind but they make redoing your face, reading and wearing contacts difficult—bits of retained oil can blur vision for a time. Petroleum jelly functions as a back-up remover.

15. *Loose, Translucent Powder.* Powder comes in light, medium and dark tones. Choose the one closest to your skin color. It should add finish, not change the color of your makeup.

16. *Lip Pencil.* Lip pencils are imperative for you who wish a sharp finish, who alter your natural liplines, and anyone whose lip color travels away from the lips in tiny wrinkles. The pencil color you seek is identical to your lipstick color. Test lip pencil with lipstick on your inner arm before buying. Color right? How's the texture? It should be firm enough to draw a clean line, not so hard it pulls the skin.

17. *Lip Brush.* Small and flat with tapered bristles, a lip brush is used to control your lipline, increase lipstick's staying time, conserve lipstick and to empty half-empty

tubes of lipstick and lipgloss. Keep it covered between uses.

18. *Lipstick*. Your type of lip protection and ideas of beauty change with age. Lipstick is a tinted gloss for the young, a stained gloss for early adulthood and opaque for later adulthood. Colors should be from your reds or skintones, but never lighter than your mouth. Avoid frosts unless you're a T-4. One lipstick color will go with everything you wear since all your reds are interrelated. Find your becoming color and *enjoy*.

19. *Lip Gloss* (optional). This shine-maker comes in pot or tub. It is used in-place-of or over lipstick—should never be considered if your lipstick bleeds.

20. *Spray Bottle of Water*. Choose any attractive bottle which sprays a fine mist. Fill with distilled or mineral water. Keep it with your cosmetics.

21. *Cotton Balls*.

22. *Cotton-Tipped Swabs*.

23. *Facial Blotting Tissues* (optional). These tissues are little linen squares in pocket packs. You press them on your face to pick up oil and moisture—made for those with oily skin.

24. *Tissues*.

25. *Brushes*. Choose flat brushes with tapered edge for eye shadow, round fat brush with tapered top for powder.

26. *Your Facial-Chart-Covered Photo*.

Note: Buy the smallest samples of new-to-you products and test colors with dimestore versions. Only invest when you're positive.

Makeup Supplies (clockwise from bottom-center) round sponge, foundation, foundation's lid, blemish coverup in tube, cream blusher, eyebrow brush/lash comb, eyebrow pencil, cotton balls, cotton-tipped swabs, tissues, eyecolor brushes, powdered eyecolor, pencil eyecolor, eyelash curler, mascara, water-sprayer, powder, powder brush, lip pencil, lipstick.

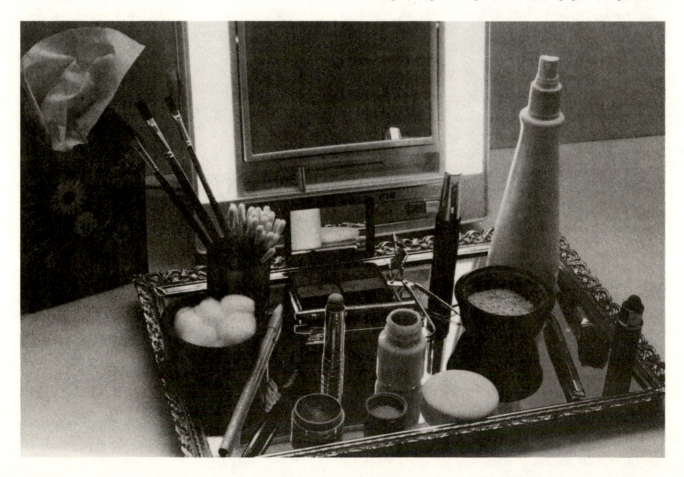

— APPLICATION —

Adapt the following techniques to your face, products, and dexterity, but apply your selections in this order.

On a clean, moisturized face, with brows neatly plucked, apply:

Foundation: Shake container; open. Mold a thin slice of sponge around your fingertip. Dip it into the foundation in container's lid (you get less this way and less is better). Dot foundation sparingly on forehead, cheeks, nose and chin. Pat/stroke it in, working *downward* with your face's contour, not upward as you do when applying moisturizer. Dip again for a second coating for under-eye and lip areas if you have dark circles or your lipstick bleeds.

Your skin should look smooth—no sign of this application. No foundation on neck, either, to smudge the inside of collars.

Blemish Coverup: Dot or brush it onto areas needing concealment or lightening. Press the area repeatedly with a gentle finger, as though you are pushing the concealer through the skin. Don't rub! Repeat until both concealer and blemish disappear.

Brush your upper lipline with concealer if your lipstick bleeds. Press till it disappears.

Should you have bags under your eyes, lift them out by brushing coverup in the valley below the curve.

If your nose is short or crooked, brush concealer down the middle from brows to tip.

Blusher: How about grinning into the mirror? Can you grin bigger? Great. Put small dots of blusher right in the middle of both "apples" your cheeks form when you grin. Relax. Now look at your Facial Photo Chart and place 2 dots to correspond with the spots on your cheeks. You're doing fine.

On your facial chart sketch a blusher pattern that begins with your dot and goes upward and outward. Those with narrow faces may design a more horizontal band of color. Those with round faces a more vertical. Play with shapes until you like what you've drawn.

Now, back to your cheeks. Place 2 more dots on each cheek extending the color in the direction your drawing indicates. Pat the dots until they blend together and feather out to nothingness on the edges.

Check your blusher against the following rules: Cheek color begins below and nearly even with the outside of the eye and extends slightly upwards, along the cheekbone to the hairline. It never enters the under-eye hollow nor approaches the nose. It doesn't go higher than the brow nor lower than the tip of the nose. Color belongs on the sides of the face, not clown-circles in front.

How did you do?

When you're happy with your glowing cheeks, you might consider a touch of blusher on forehead, chin or even the sides of your jaw (if it needs contouring). Remember that red acts like a darker shading and makes the items it touches recede . . . but keep it subtle.

Fashion switches from pale to semi-bright, from rosy apples to shadowed hollows, so watch magazine covers to see how blusher is used today. You want an individual style, but modification can keep it contemporary.

Eye-Makeup Foundation: If you use it, place the tiniest amount on fingertip or cotton-tipped swab. Dot each eyelid and underbrow area (1 dab makes 4 dots). Blend over entire underbrow area, down to your lashes. Blend gently.

Brow Brush: Brush brows straight up as though they were electrified. Then brush outward making a line of the uppermost hairs.

Eyebrow Pencil: Draw tiny hairs wherever they're needed to complete your best brow shape. Use two colors if one isn't natural enough. Check your Facial Chart for confirmation of the look you've drawn. If brows don't stay in place, touch them lightly with moustache wax.

Eyeshadows: To work wonders transforming your imperfectly-proportioned eyes into excitingly beautiful ones, use eyeshadows. Look at your eyes in your Facial Chart; note which parts of your eye area are too thick,

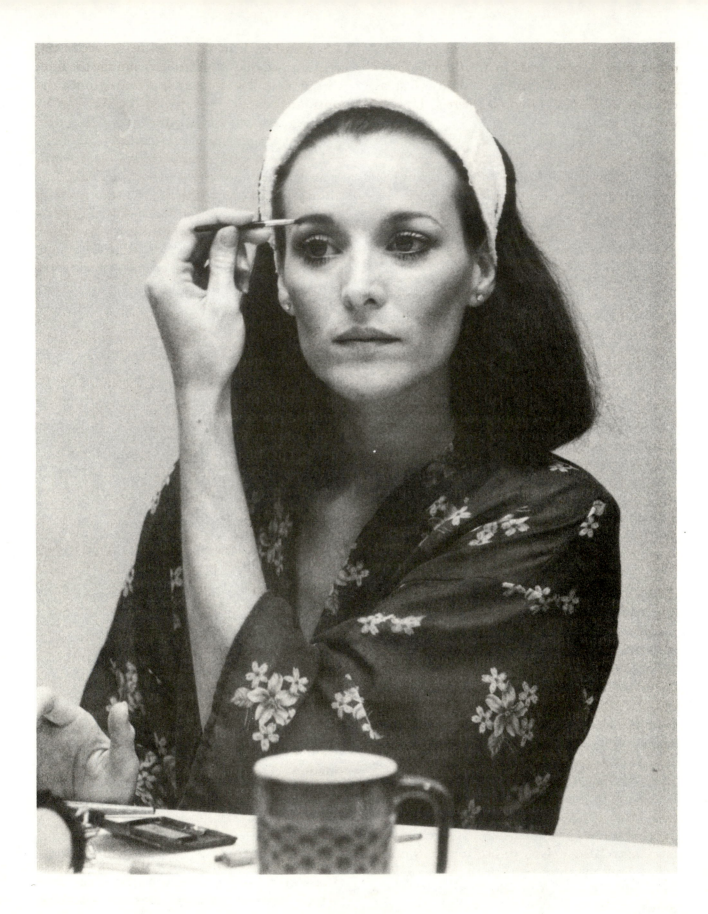

T-1 applying makeup

thin, straight or droopy; "X" areas to be corrected. Label those areas in your chart's margin. Dark and light shadow contour eye areas without appearing phony. Here's how it works.

If your eyes are wide-set, use a darker shadow in the area between eyelid/peak of brow/side of nose. Circle this area on your Facial chart and mark it "darker." Experiment with a darker skintone shadow in the same area on your face. You'll notice less space between your eyes. Keep the most intense color near the inner corner of the eye, and never extend color beyond the outer corner. Dust pressed eyeshadow onto your lids or underbrow area with a brush or apply cream shadow with the tip of your finger or a cotton-tipped swab. Use the swab to smudge and blend-away all lines of demarcation.

For narrow-set eyes, sweep a darker shadow up and outward beyond the outer corner of the eye. You might also experiment using a lighter color on either side of your nose, just above the tear ducts. Note how your eyes appear to move apart. Mark your chart with the areas and notations of "lighter" or "darker."

Prominent eyelids can be minimized with darker shadow on the lid-to-crease area.

Thin-to-invisible eyelids can be maximized with a light, bright shadow on lid . . . use one of your lighter, brighter *neutrals*.

Deep-set eyes should have a light shadow in the above-the-eye-crease to bring the area forward.

Shallow eye sockets can appear deeper with a smudged dark line in the crease where a shadow would fall.

Always smudge eyeshadow so it is indistinct and shadowy. You want to look as though you grew that way, not that you applied makeup.

Eyeliner: Pencil eyeliners are particularly handy. Accent perfect eyes with sidewise V brackets at the start and end of each eye. These should be as close to the lash as you can work and extend up to 1/4 inch along upper and lower lashes, leaving an unlined space in the center to display your lashes. Smudge the line.

If your eyes are close-set, line only the *outside* of upper and lower lashes.

For wide-set eyes, line only the *inner* edges of upper and lower lashes.

Down-sloping eyes can appear straight with a dark, smudged eyeliner extending outward in a normal curve where your eyes turn downwards. There should be no lightness between the curve you've drawn and your eye. Try this first on your Facial Chart overlay. When you've worked out a design you like, try it on yourself.

When using a liquid eyeliner, apply it in dots as close to the lash as possible. Smudge dots with a cotton-tipped swab. Eyeliner makes lashes look full and thick.

In general, use a neutral color on your lids, a darker tone in the crease, and a lighter tint on the browbone.

Eyelash Curler: Turn nearly-invisible upper lashes into visible curving ones with an eyelash curler. To use: look straight ahead. Lay the opened curler against your cheek with upper lashes between the rubber sections. Gently close. Assert pressure, release, press, release—three times. Slip curler further out on the same lash and repeat. Now, curl your other upper lash. Using the eyelash curler *before* you add mascara cuts down lash breakage and eliminates mascara buildup in the instrument.

Mascara: Warm tube or bottle by rolling it several times between your palms. Extract the wand and let it dry for a few moments if you have the time. Then, holding the wand horizontally and with your chin against your neck, looking down, brush down on both upper lashes. Turning wand vertically and lifting your chin, brush across lashes from side to side. Let them dry a bit, then comb through lashes to eliminate clumping. Next, dipping wand as needed, repeatedly brush from base to tip of upper lashes. Using wand's tip, work lashes outward if your eyes are close-set, upward if your eyes are wide-set.

For extra thickness, brush baby powder onto lashes with a tiny tooth brush. Repeat your mascara application. Comb again.

Tilt your head down as you brush the tips of your lower lashes with the wand held vertically. Slip a folded tissue under your lower lashes and lift them up, blotting excess mascara from the underside to eliminate potential smudging.

Cake mascara takes more time than the wand, but it allows additional control and is less likely to bleed. Practice when results aren't important. You'll be a master when results are *everything*.

Mascara Remover: To remove mascara—wet a cottonball in eye-makeup remover, close your eye, and stroke downward several times. Open eye and gently stroke outward, underneath your eye. Repeat if necessary. Cleanse other eye area.

Powder: Dip a fresh cottonball into loose powder, shake off the excess, then fluff the remainder onto your face. Lightly dust away visible powder with a powder brush. Always brush down so as not to raise the tiny hairs on your face. Powder supplies a matte finish and sets your makeup.

Lip Pencil: Check your Facial Chart for an ideal lip shape, then draw that design on your mouth with a lip pencil. Begin at the center and draw the lines outward. It helps to steady your hand by bracing a curled little finger against your chin. Correct outline errors until it pleases you.

If your lips are uneven in width, line only the thicker one and use a darker-toned lipstick on it. Use a lighter brighter color on the unlined, thinner lip.

Lip Brush: Brush lipstick inside the penciled outline in an up-and-down manner, not side-to-side. Carefully cover your penciled line but don't extend beyond it. And don't blot your lips! Lipstick no longer needs blotting and doing so ruins your finish.

If lipstick wears off too quickly or bleeds up the fine lines above your upper lip, dust lips lightly with powder before applying pencil or lipstick and more powder before a second application of color. If your lipstick still runs, throw away all frosted or glossy lipsticks, moisturize the lip area much more than you're doing, and thin the surrounding area at least weekly. Moisturize at night.

Lip Gloss: If worn over lipstick, lip gloss should be dotted on the center of upper and lower lip, not carried to the corners of the mouth. Tracing a full mouth with gloss will blur your carefully drawn lipline. If gloss is used alone, it can be worn on the entire mouth. Apply with a lipbrush. Lip gloss with sunscreen is perfect for beach or ski slope for women of all ages.

Never reshape your lips if you intend to wear gloss alone. Corrections will show.

Check Point: Recheck your blush, your eyes, the overall look of you. Retouch if necessary. Less is better than too much, so begin with a light hand and work up to more dramatic techniques for more dramatic occasions. Do your makeup carefully and properly each time and both technique and speed will increase. Besides, you'll always look wonderful.

Spray Bottle of Water: As the last movement before leaving your cosmetic area, lightly mist your face to set the makeup. Never mist the eye area unless your mascara is waterproof. This misting can be repeated whenever your face needs reviving. Try it. You'll like it.

— MAKEUP PROTECTION —

Bacteria enjoys many of your makeup products, so don't share them with anyone or use saliva to moisten products. Wash your hands before applying anything to your face; wipe screwtops with tissue before replacing lids; soak sponges and brushes in warm water with mild soap or Woolite® (rinse, then dry brushes with bristles up); keep containers tightly closed; and discard any product which becomes discolored, changes odor, or loses it consistency (becomes thinner or thicker).

Since mascara is particularly susceptible to contamination, use not more than two mascaras at any time and keep others sealed until the first are empty.

If your eyes or eyelids become infected, discontinue all eye-makeup products for at least ten days after irritation disappears. Then reintroduce products individually until the culprit is discovered. If your problem is an allergic reaction, and not contamination, make a note in the back of this book: Never use "_____" again.

— EXTRA MAKEUP TIPS —

Eyelash Dyeing: Dyeing your eyelashes can temporarily replace mascara, but dye must be applied by a professional. Never attempt dyeing when eyelids are irritated or puffy or if you have indications of allergies. The entire process takes ten minutes and causes only minor discomfort unless eyes are unusually sensitive. If your skin isn't oily and you stay out of the sun, your dye-job should last a month. Oil dissolves the tint and sunlight bleaches it. Major advantage of dyed lashes is looking scrubbed-face super for a special trip (honeymoon?).

For Travel: Keep 2 clear-plastic, zippered envelopes packed and in your travel case.

One envelope to contain small amounts of all indispensable makeup items. Collect product samples and/or transfer makeup from your larger containers into tiny ones.

The second envelope to be filled with comb, shampoo, skin cleansing and moisturizing products, toothbrush and paste, bath salts and perfume—all the overnight supplies you can't be without.

With these envelopes refilled at the *close* of each trip, you'll be ready to go at the drop of an invitation.

During Hot Weather: When temperatures soar above eighty-five degrees, refrigerate your makeup. Heat causes disintegration.

For Photographs: Avoid black liner and mascara. Substitute a softer color.

When Fashion Changes: Visit your cosmetic department and ask to have a makeup demonstration. You already understand your

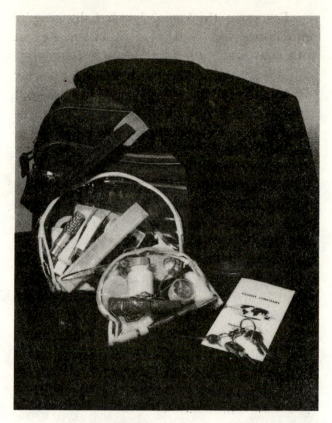

Travel Envelopes

face and what can or should be done with it, but a cosmetician can add the look of "today." Keep an open mind and update colors and application methods *whenever they're better than your own.* Two years is maximum for any single look.

Glasses Wearers: You have unique eye makeup concerns. Lenses for the far-sighted magnify your features and will broadcast mistakes in application techniques or color selection. Check your finished makeup with glasses in place and correct if necessary.

Lenses for the near-sighted shrink apparent eye size, so you'll need a more dramatic presentation and every trick you can locate to make your eyes look larger.

Because of their major impact, glasses have their own chapter. It follows next.

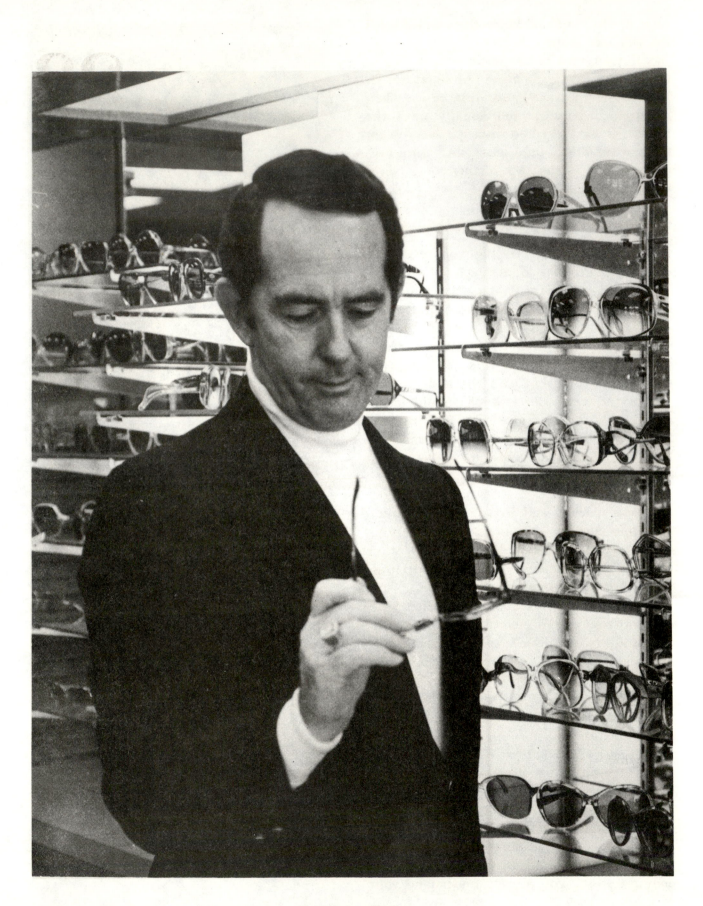

T-4 selecting glasses

23

Your Glasses

The saying, "Men never make passes . . . . ," is untrue. You've proven that. Glasses can be fun. They are, additionally, your most important accessory.

Glasses correct faulty vision, shield eyes from glare and/or add a personal signature as do the oversized frames that identify Jacqueline Onassis. But, choose them carefully, or the image of YOU will be sabotaged.

No other accessory is so instantly noticeable. Glasses improve your facial shape, function as instant makeup, perk up your wardrobe, and finish your look. Dark glasses add the further pluses of aiding your vision in bright light, cutting glare, and reducing unattractive squint lines.

That's a lot for your money, but how do you avoid mistakes? *Be informed and choose carefully.*

When selecting dark glasses, you'll be faced with six choices of lens not counting the various tints or the materials (glass or plastic) of which they're made.

1. *Polarized Lens* is excellent. It's a laminate of seven layers: one which filters-out ninety-eight percent of the horizontal light, two which block ninety-six percent of ultraviolet light, and four which lend shatter and scratch resistance. This lens is inexpensive and practical—universally fine for hard-to-block glare such as you'll find boating, fishing or snow skiing.

2. *Mirror Lens* is also effective eye protection since it reflects light and glare, but it's anti-social. No one enjoys talking to a person with invisible eyes.

3. *Photochromic or Light-Adjusting Lens* is a good choice for ducking in-and-out but not for wear in your car. It needs the ultraviolet light which doesn't penetrate car windows to trigger a color change. You have the choice of darker or lighter photochromic lenses—those that go from dark to medium or from medium to light. None cover the full range of potential lighting problems.

4. *Gradient Lens* is tinted differently across the face of the lens. In some glasses it's lighter at the bottom and darker on top to allow for easier reading. In others the tint varies from side-to-side. This lens is stylish but inadequate for glare.

5. *One Color Lens* was once your only choice and now it's less effective than the mirrored or polarized. Light tints give little protection; darker tones are moderate safeguards.

6. *Mirrored-Photochromic Lens* is said to be good for all glare conditions. It's amber on overcast days, turns brown on sunny days and gray for peak protection on cold, brilliant days. The precision-ground lenses are made from optical glass and treated for impact resistance. Check their weight and the amount of distraction the mirroring causes viewers.

If dark glasses are to lend protection, they must be so dark your eyes are nearly invisible. A deep smoke or neutral gray is the best choice, followed by dark sage green, then amber.

Function is a first consideration even though buying solely for visual effect is tempting.

Check lenses for distortion. Hold them above your head and turn the lenses until you catch reflections from overhead lights on the inside. Slightly rotate them. The faintest distortion or blemish will be apparent. Flawed lenses can be annoying at best and harmful to your eyes at worst.

Check the frames for strength. Twist them gently. You need assurance they'll last for years, not proof that mistreatment will shatter them.

Check the fit at the nose bridge. Rotate your head, look up and down, try to dislodge them.

Check the fit at the sides. Glasses should be snug but comfortable at your temples and top of your ears. Have them adjusted if they hurt.

Frames should cover your brows and be at least the width of your face.

Choose a frame color that coordinates with the tint of your lens (if it's tinted), your Type and your coloring.

T-1 Frames are round, rounded or petal-shaped. Best choice is a plastic that is similar to hair color. If it's tortoiseshell, choose as little striation as possible. Dark glasses can have any of your bright or neutral Becoming Colors, but an *only* pair should be conservative.

T-2 Frames are oval plastic, your haircolor, or soft taupe, gray, mauve, plum or lavender. Look for frames with indistinct coloration—a mere suggestion of tone. If the oval shape doesn't flatter, choose frames with arching lines or geometrics with softened corners. Avoid the gimicky, stark, heavy, bright and those with diamond chips or monograms.

T-3 Frames have angular shapes such as squares, rectangles, multi-sided with semi-softened edges, aviator—frames with apparent weight and authority. Tortoise is perfect in either its dark or light forms. Match them to your hair. The copper and bronze metallics can also be effective. Avoid bright colors and cute trims.

T-4 Frames are ovalized plastic the color of your hair or silver-gray. Another choice is silver metal in a becoming shape. Choose a sleek or high-fashion style—nothing heavy, textured, bright or ornamented.

Match frame size and weight to your scale. Heroic features are balanced by large glasses, delicate features by small.

Select frames also by your facial shape.

Oval has the widest choice in glasses. Enjoy!

Round is enhanced by wider-than-high frames with elliptical or softened angles. Low-placed side-bars are flattering.

Long needs width above the eye and sufficient depth to reach the center of the cheek.

Square is softened by rounded or elongated ovals.

Heart seeks width below the eyes—styles which lend width to the cheek area, diminish the forehead.

Triangle and *Diamond* like rounded lines with width above the eyes.

Consider facial irregularities:

High Forehead is balanced with oval curves below the eye.

Close-set Eyes are widened with frames that are tinted darker at the outside and are clear or neutral at the bridge of the nose.

Wide-set Eyes or those with *Thick Noses* reverse the procedure. Their frames are best dark at the center and light at the sides.

Long Nose is shortened with wide frames having a high-riding bridge.

Short Nose is lengthened with a low-bridged round or rectangular frame.

Fashion frames with high or low temple bars often improve peripheral vision. But avoid extreme materials, shapes and trims. YOU're the star, not your glasses.

Wow, how do you assimilate all of the above?

Pull out your facial photo once again, overlay it with tracing paper, and sketch a pair of glasses which incorporate all of the previously-mentioned ideas that pertain to you. Or sketch several pairs before making a composite that includes the best of each. Take your sketch with you when you glasses-shop to save time and frustration. You may never find the glasses of your sketch, but you'll be better able to judge available compromises.

Those needing bifocals may prefer multi-focal lenses which have no telltale line across the lower section. But be certain the one you're considering offers a sufficiently wide reading strip for general use, that you can safely navigate stairs in them, and that they won't be relegated to sole use as "restaurant" glasses.

Keep abreast of changes in eyewear. Old glasses can date you as neatly as an old hairdo.

Save money on prescription dark glasses by having same-shape frames for both dark and daily. Clear plastic prescription lenses can be inexpensively dyed, so dye your next-to-latest lenses and insert them into the dark frames. Repeat whenever you change prescriptions.

Wear dark glasses only when you're outdoors unless you've chosen the photochromic type. Indoors, dark glasses block light too much—will harm your vision eventually.

Glasses are available in plastic or glass lenses. Plastic is light but requires extra care to keep unscratched. Glass doesn't scratch but it's heavy—may slip down your nose.

Wash glasses daily with detergent and warm water. Polish them dry with a soft cloth (his old handkerchief?). Keep them safe in their case when not in use.

Contact Lenses eliminate glasses-selection problems as well as visual handicaps. But watch their color. Have them tinted the exact tone of your iris, not a bright blue, or green, or brown. You have perfect coloring—don't imbalance it with an eye color that isn't you.

Some safety tips include: avoid wearing your *contacts* in the barber or beauty shop where hairspray and nailpolish vapors are in the air, and avoid using sprays at home when your contacts are in place. Carefully cleanse your hands of soap, shampoo and aftershave or fragrance before inserting contacts.

Insert soft contacts before you apply makeup, hard lenses, after. Be aware that wrinkles can be caused by contacts—too much squinting and manipulation of the eye area.

Finally, comparison shop for glasses or contacts as you do for your clothing. The same frames will often be available at more than one store and for more than one price.

Have you found a fragrance as perfect for you as your new glasses? If not, don't miss the next chapter . . .

24

Your Fragrance

Subtle scent—lifting spirits like a breeze off the sea, swirling round like a silken shawl, fulfilling, delighting, teasing, awakening passion, or overpowering, disagreeable, Eau de Gymsox, the right cologne on the wrong person—*which will it be for you?*

Natural body scent plays an erotic role in the animal kingdom. Could it enhance human sexuality? Scientists aren't sure, but who wants to test it? Body odor is culturally unacceptable, and most of man's original sensitivity to scent has been lost. Deodorized, man waits on the perfumer to complete him.

Information can increase your fragrance pleasure, decrease your potential problems and help you escape the whim of your Christmas stocking. It follows.

— YOUR SENSE OF SMELL —

The sense of smell has priority over sight, sound, taste and touch. It alone hot-lines a message from nose to brain with no intermediaries. Each waking moment 20 to 40 million odor-sensors (olfactory recepters) are at work sending signals at speeds faster than that of sound. Assessment and cataloguing of scents are carried out so rapidly you're unaware of the process.

Smells can linger in olfactory memory for a lifetime yet be recalled instantly with accompanying emotions intact. One whiff of *Avon®* lipstick and I'm eight years old; it's Halloween; and *I'm wearing lipstick.*

Sally will always react to *Old Spice Aftershave*. Bob wore it constantly. Now *that* scent on passing males makes her physically ill even though it's been years since he jilted her. And she used to love it!

— PERFUME'S HISTORY —

Early perfumes were either strong or extravagantly used. Primitive tribes had scents potent enough to kill every fly in a modern football stadium. Cleopatra so perfumed the sails of her barge that they were scented before they could be sighted. Napolean Bonaparte used 2 bottles of cologne a day!

Today's perfumes can be lighter than yesteryear's since bathing facilities are more available and personal hygiene is practiced. So a word of warning . . . no educated person's scent should precede him nor linger after he is gone.

Dramatic changes in modern perfumes come from two sources: chemistry laboratories and the young.

Sophisticated, synthetic fragrances now enhance major perfumes giving "noses," experts who spend years blending hundreds of scents into one perfume, many more fragrances to choose from.

Young people, less culturally circumscribed than their parents and aware of ecology, have spotlighted "natural" scents and incorporated them into daily living. Credit them with the huge success of civet, ambergris and musk. Adults have adopted these "naturals" in the fluid form but also as perfumed candles and incense.

— MALE AND FEMALE REACTION TO SCENT —

Scent is no longer a woman's province.

Men choose scent to underline their masculinity, feel well-groomed, appear successful and sometimes to arouse the female.

Since males annually spend over a billion dollars for toiletries and nearly 80% of these funds go for after-shaves and colognes, they obviously like it for themselves. How do they feel about a woman's use of fragrance?

Most men prefer their women to be perfumed. When a well-known magazine asked men if fragrance improved their sex life the answers were affirmative. One male commented, "The smell of a woman wearing a nice fragrance can be very appealing and sexy"; another stated, "Fragrance instantly puts sexual ideas into my head"; and a third said, "I'd fall in love with just about anyone wearing *Shalimar*."

Christian Dior once said, "Feminity is inconceivable without the association of fragrance. When I recall a charming woman, her fragrance is an inseparable part of the memory."

Women choose scent to feel feminine, enjoy the fragrance, feel successful and assured, draw compliments and attract both men and women.

Mlle. Gabrielle Chanel, French designer, stated, "Perfume is a vital part of the success of a woman; without perfume no elegance is possible."

With keener noses than men's, women instantly detect and involuntarily judge a person's odor, a strong influence toward accepting or rejecting that person. Be warned, odor is *all* important when a female detects another woman's scent on her man's clothes or person . . . perfume tattles.

— CASE FOR THE SINGLE SCENT —

Once, each lady and gentleman chose one fragrance as a lifetime signature. A single fragrance would pervade person, hair, clothing. Spouse, children, lovers, friends forever associated a certain scent with a particular person. One whiff of *Lily of the Valley* and Caroline was instantly recalled.

Today you wear those colognes you see advertised, you like on others, or you're given for your birthday. Fickle, you may change fragrance weekly, daily, twice a day, by mood, by activity, by habit. You succeed in missing perfume's full potential.

Single Scent identification of an individual is immediate, emotional and invaluable. I love wearing just one perfume . . . my "trademark" scent. Others look for me when *my* fragrance wafts past. My clothes and closet reflect it. I repeat the perfume with sachet, dusting powder, lotion and purse spray . . . am gifted with it in ever-new forms. Nice.

Anne Fogarty recommended the single scent. She called it your "One Scent Stamp."

Want a Single Scent for yourself? I'm glad you do even though locating that special fragrance may not be easy. Like searching for the perfect mate, you may have to flirt with many before finding one that clicks.

— SELECTING YOUR SIGNATURE SCENT —

There are three criteria: it must reinforce your type, smell good on your skin, and last at least four hours.

The perfect scent will reinforce your personality, coloring, and physical characteristics and make your confidence soar. Animated young-at-hearts will seek a light, citrus or green scent. Romantics want a warm, delicate, sweetly complex fragrance or a single flower such as lavender or violet. Earthy types should smell richly opulent, sultry, earthy, mysterious or exotic. Classic sophisticates seek a cool, expensively modern signature.

To simplify your search I've grouped many of today's name brand perfumes into four groups. Look for them beginning on page 142. Male and female divisions are for convenience not exclusivity, so if you like a scent marketed for the opposite sex, wear it.

It must smell good on your skin. Perfume isn't complete until it is applied to the skin and one's body chemistry acts upon it. A scent on you will smell differently than it does from the bottle or on anyone else.

It must last at least four hours. Are you one of the unfortunates on whom fragrance disappears? Perhaps you can change that. High altitude, dry air and cool weather suppress scent, but you needn't move from Denver. Some fragrances have longer-lasting ingredients than others, and the perfumes, creams, solids and oils in each scent collection will stay on the longest. Try them!

1. Stop by a perfume or men's cologne counter some morning when you are wearing *no* fragrance. Morning, because your nose is most sensitive then; no fragrance, for you want an accurate test.

2. Try two or at most three of the perfumes displayed. The testers are there for exactly that purpose. Your nose can't differentiate more than three scents at a time.

3. Dab a few drops of your first sample on the inside of your right wrist. Ask the salesperson or a friend to rub it in. Repeat on your left wrist with a second sample. Repeat in the crook of one elbow for the third.

4. Don't sniff any perfumes from the bottle. Wait for a few seconds after a scent has been applied . . . now take a whiff. Keep perfume off your hands and off the tip of your nose when you test aromas.

5. Check all three scents and note your reactions in a notebook. Some scents you may love, or hate. If one's so unpleasant you can't stand it, scrub your wrist with soap and water and record your reaction in appropriate language. You'd hate to try it again!

6. Check all test areas again in thirty minutes. Record your results.

7. Check again after two hours. record.

8. Check again at four hours after application. A scent shouldn't be expected to perform longer, but you'd expect it to go the full round.

9. Wait a day before you test again. Time refreshes your nose.

10. Discard all poor performers before testing your winners, two at a time. Reduce your selection to your BEST scent.

11. Buy a small bottle of this fragrance. Use generously. Reapply every four hours. Collect reactions of others. If compliments fail to follow, try your second choice in the same manner.

12. Congratulations! You've found your Signature Scent. Now to use it properly.

— HOW TO USE PERFUME —

Let's begin with the cautions:

Don't ... *wear scent when sunbathing.* Sunlight on perfume can cause skin discoloration, irritation, conflict with the fragrance of tanning lotions, and, like your left-over lunch, draw flies.

... *put scent on your furs.* Scent may discolor them.

... *put scent into plastic containers.* Fragrance can alter.

... *expose fragrance to sunlight, bright light, heat or excessive age.* Scent is delicate, the alcohol will evaporate and the essences change in composition.

... *put scent behind your ears.* That's wasteful. There are better places.

... *combine scents.* Use the same in all its forms.

Do ... *spray or rub fragrance onto pulse points:* temples, below the jawline, behind the knees, inside of ankles, at insteps, at warm creases. *Body heat is needed to activate scent.*

... *apply after-shave, cologne and scented lotion* to damp skin if fragrance fails to linger. Buff it in. Moist skin holds more scent than dry.

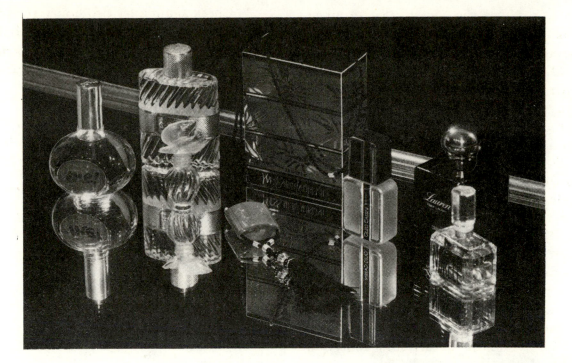

Containers can be Typed as well as the fragrance within them. from left to right: T-1 fragrance & bottle, T-2 fragrances & bottles, T-3 fragrances, box, pendant & bottle, T-3 bottle with T-1 fragrance & cap (an example of poor coordination), T-4 fragrance and bottle.

... *choose perfume* over cologne or toilet water when you need more potent, long-lasting results, need a finishing touch, and can afford the most expensive form of scent.

... *choose Eau de Toilette*, or toilet water, when you wish a less intense fragrance or a scent background.

... *choose Eau de Cologne*, or cologne, lightest of all, as an all-over spray refresher (consider transferring it into a dime-store atomizer), as a back or foot rub, in your final hair or lingerie rinse, on a blotter in your stationery box, on your drawer lining paper, on your pillow cases, and on air-conditioner grids or light bulbs (for more fragrant rooms).

... *choose spray purse flacon* for refreshing your scent when away from home.

... *choose solid perfume*, longer lasting than liquids and available in compacts, lockets, rings and bracelets.

... *choose cream sachet* for dry or peeling skins. Formulated without alcohol, it's soothing.

... *choose dry sachet* (for bureau drawers, inside luggage or inside purses (empty perfume bottles and bars of scented soap make admirable substitutes).

... *choose bath oil* if your fragrance fails to cling, to rub on skin before showering or to perfume your bath water.

... *choose dusting powder and talc* to absorb after-bath moisture or to sprinkle between the bedsheets on a humid evening.

... *choose scented candles* for spreading "your" fragrance throughout your room or apartment.

Enjoy your fragrance in all its forms, but remember—perfume that is delicate outdoors, in a cool room, or on a cool body can be overpowering on a heated body or inside a packed elevator. Switch to lighter scents in the summer.

Fragrances to try if you're active, young-at-heart, animated, a party-person—a T-1.	

—HERS—

Arden's "Blue Grass,"	Guerlain's "Eau de Guerlain," "Ode"
Balmaine's "Jolie Madame"	"Calvin Klein"
Geoffery Beene's "Red"	Ralph Lauren's "Lauren"
Bonne Bell's "Bonnie"	Love's "Daisy L"
Burrows' "Stephen B"	Matchabelli's "Aviance," "Cachet"
Carven's "Ma Griffe"	Monteil's "Germaine"
"Charles of the Ritz"	Nestle-LeMur's "Whisper"
Chanel's "Chanel 19"	"Molly Parnis"
"Christalle"	Revlon's "Charlie"
Coty's "Muguet des Bois"	Ricci's "Cappricci"
"Smitty"	Shulton's "Blue Jeans"
"Oscar de la Renta"	Ultima II's "Ciara"
Dior's "Miss Dior"	Weil's "Antilope," "Weil de Weil"
Faberge's "Woodhue"	YSL's "Rive Gauche"
Factor's "Just Call Me Maxi"	

—HIS—

Aramis' "Devon"	Faberge's "Woodhue"
"900 Herbal	Givenchy's "Gentlemen"
Arden's "Sandalwood"	Jovan's "Grass Oil for Men"
Balenciaga's "Ho Hang"	Lauren's "Polo"
Beene's "Grey Flannel"	Lord Byron's "20 Lengths"
"British Sterling"	Revlon's "Chaz"
Caron's "Pour Un Homme"	"Royal Pub"
Chanel's "Chanel for Men"	Rorer Int.'s "Old Spice"
Coureges' "Eau de Toilette"	Swank's "Royal Copenhagen"
Dior's "Eau Savage"	"Serrano"
English Leather's "Bitter Lemon,"	William's "Mon Triomphe"
"Timberline"	
"Wind Drift"	

Fragrances to try if you're romantic, creative, sensitive and gentle—a T-2.	

—HERS—

Arden's "Cabriole," "Memoire Cherie"	Guerlain's "Charmade," "L'Heure Bleue,"
Avon's "Patchwork"	"Parure"
Balenciaga's "Le De," "Quadrille"	Houbigant's "Essence Rare," "Quelques Fleurs"
Bouchard's "Mon Bonheur"	Jovan's "Mink & Pearls," "Woman"
Caron's "Infini," "Narcisse Noir"	Lagerfield's "Chloe"
Chanel's "Chanel #22"	Lanvin's "Arpege," "My Sin"
"Cie"	La Roche's "Fidgi"
Coty's "Lily of the Valley," "L'Origan,"	Lauder's "Youth Dew," "Estee"
"Masumi"	Matchabelli's "Wind Song"
D'Albret's "Ecusson"	Revlon's "Jontue"
deMarkoff's "Enigma"	Ricci's "L'Air du Temps"
Dior's "Diorissimo"	Shulton's "Desert Flower"
Evyan's "Most Precious," "White Shoulders"	Worth's "Je Reviens"
Faberge's "Flambeau"	Yardley's "English Lavender"
"Gucci Parfum "1"	

—HIS—

Alexander de Markoff's "Aston"
"Eau de Balenciaga"
"Bill Blass"
Evyan's "The Baron"
Faberge's "Aphrodisia," "Zizanie"
Guerlain's "Habit Rouge," "Vetiver"

Gucci's "Pour Homme"
Halston's "Z-14"
Jovan's "Monsieur Jovan," "Man"
Lord Byron's "Eman"
Yardley's "English Lavender"
YSL's "YSL for Men"

—HERS—

Avon's "Unspoken"
Coty's "Emeraude," "Wild Musk"
Dana's "Ambush," "Tabu"
Deprez's "Bal a Versailles"
Dior's "Fleur Savage"
Faberge's "Babe," "Tigress"
Guerlain's "Charmade," "Mitsouko," "Shalimar"
Hermes' "Amazone"
Houbigant's "Ambergris Oil,"
    "Civit Oil," "Musk Oil"
Jovan's "Frankencense & Myrh"
    "Ginseng," "Musk Oil"
Myrugia's "Orgia"

Nestle-LeMur's "Balalaika,"
    "Indiscret," "Sirroco"
Patou's "Amour Amour"
Pucci's "Vivara"
Revlon's "Intimate"
Ricci's "Farouche"
Rubenstein's "Heaven Sent"
Scannon's "Tabac Blond"
Shiseida's "Zen"
Weil's "Zibeline"
Worth's "Je Reviens"
YSL's "Opium"

—HIS—

Bell's "Colorado Sage"
Byron's "Mink Oil"
Cochran's "Pierre Cardin"
Coty's "Ginseng for Men"
    "Musk for Men," "Sex Appeal for Men"
Dana's "Canoe"
Dior's "Eau Savage"
English Leather's "Musk Cologne for Men"
Faberge's "Brute," "Macho"
"Hai Karate"

Halston's "Z-14"
Houbigant's "Musk"
Jovan's "Musk for Men"
    "Ginseng for Men," "Monsier Jovan"
Lentheric's "Tweed"
Rabanne's "Pour L'Homme"
Revlon's "Braggi," "Black Tie," "Roman Brio"
"Russian Leather"
Swank's "Jade East"

Fragrances to try if you're cool, classic, elegant, sophisticated—a T-4.

—HERS—

Caron's "Nuit de Noel"
Chanel's "Chanel #5"
Chas/Ritz's "Ritz"
Corday's "Toujours Moi"
Coty's "Elan," "Imprevu,"
    "L'Aimant," "Nuance"
Dana's "20 Carats"
Dior's "Diorella"
"Givenchy III"
Faberge's "Aphrodisia"
Guerlain's "Imperiale"
"Halston"
Klein's "Blazer"

Lagerfeld's "Chloe"
Lauder's "Aliage," "Azuree"
    "Private Collection"
Millot's "Crepe de Chine"
"Norell"
Patou's "Joy"
Pucci's "Miss Zadig"
Rabanne's "Calandre"
Rubenstein's "Courant"
Schiaparelli's "Shocking"
"Irma Shorell"
Shisedo's "Inoui"
YSL's "Y"

—HIS—

"Aramis"
"Bogart"
"Chanel for Men"
Faberge's "Musk for Men"
Guerlain's "Imperiale"
"Gucci"

Halston 1-12"
Pucci's "Signor Vivara"
Rochas's "Monsieur Rochas"
Molyneux's "Captain Molyneux"
Scannon's "Kanon"

One last warning: noses lose their sensitivity to an oft-worn scent, and temptation is great to steadily increase both amount of fragrance and frequency of application. Don't do it! You owe it to your audience to treat scent subtly. Cleopatra's day is gone.

The perfume lists are incomplete since new fragrances appear daily and those presently on the market haven't *all* been typed. These are selected to speed your research and offer a place to record your observations. Add new scents, strike off those you hate, have fun!

Does cosmetic surgery entice or revolt? Few remain neutral concerning this formerly hush-hush subject. The next two chapters may offer enlightenment, but chapter twenty five, which follows immediately, is personal—a face-lift diary.

## 25

Your Apparent Age

— A FACE-LIFT DIARY —

Turtlenecks went with everything. They had to; for although my face retained its youthful animation, its jawline vanished under loose neck muscles and crepey skin. My age? Forty-four.

I could ignore the problem most days but was faced with it each time my photographer husband used me as a model. No pose nor lighting change produced flattering negatives, and his favorite 35 mm film didn't allow touch-ups. He needed a larger camera or a different model while I needed some flattering pictures. Our solution came when an honest friend asked, "Have you considered cosmetic surgery?"

Of course not! And yet . . . my new career included both television and public appearances where lighting could be cruel. A Face Lift? Why not? What would it entail? What would it cost? Would a physician agree I needed one?

I made appointments with two well-recommended plastic surgeons. Both suggested my recent weight loss and the inherited transparency of my skin had prematurely aged me. Both recommended a Lift.

I liked both men, but they proposed two different solutions. Doctor A advised a Mini Lift plus eye surgery and a Chemical Peel of the area below my nose, excluding cheeks. Doctor B proposed an Extensive Face Lift that included lifting the sagging muscles of my face and neck with supporting sutures. He felt this would correct my droopy eyelids without surgery. Doctor B also suggested a wait of three months after surgery before determining whether a Peel was needed. Doctor B's recommendation sounded most sensible. I took the idea home to ponder.

My financial backer and husband, bless him, voiced concern over the discomfort such surgery might cause me before even mentioning the cost. Dr. B considered my husband's occupation, my budding (not yet financially productive) career, and our two children in college in setting the $1,200 fee which included all postoperative care. The hospital bill, just over $500, covered expenses for two nights plus four hours of operating room time. With the anesthesiologist, our bill totaled $2,000. Whew . . . beauty is expensive!

My surgery date was set a month in advance, and I worked like a demon to clear a six-week block on my calendar and to lose any weight I wanted lost. Doctor B said he wanted no weight loss after surgery to destroy his work. I agreed.

Before Hospital Day I had second thoughts, but a look in the mirror plus my curiosity carried me through. I really wanted to know what it was like to have a Lift.

I checked into the hospital feeling young and spry. Even though my doctor had been paid in full ten days earlier, at his request, I was startled by the hospital's request for their $500 in advance.

Later, after chest Xrays, urine and blood samples, blood pressure, and temperature were taken, I sat on my bed like a lavender paja-maed heiress. Supper was light and palatable. For the third consecutive night I shampooed my hair with a prescribed shampoo to kill all hair and scalp germs. Makeup removal exposed my familiar, if aging face. Farewell. Then into my strange bed, a Heinlein adventure for escape, surprisingly soon a sleeping pill. I closed my eyes.

Surgery Day arrived early and I was asked if I had any contact lenses, false hairpieces, false eyelashes, jewelry, money, or false teeth. Were my fingernails or toenails polished? "No" seemed to be the correct response to all questions. I was given a "groggy" pill, a rough, open-back night shirt, and a ride on a stretcher. When I awoke I was holding my husband's hand, it was afternoon, and I couldn't see.

There was, amazingly, no pain, but I didn't feel well. My head felt large and twingy and nervous tension coursed through my limbs. My hands were tied to the bedrails and my head was wrapped in a pressure bandage that would be in place for twenty-four hours. Having my nostrils and mouth free of bandage while my eyes-head-throat were covered made me less claustrophobic than I'd expected.

The first night was interminable. Sleepless, I slipped my restraints and turned over and over in bed. By morning my chin was one large blister and both elbows were raw from the rough hospital sheets. This was all unnecessary and wouldn't have occurred if I'd told Dr. B I didn't tolerate tranquilizers. After a fitful sleep, I awakened to hear my doctor speaking to me. He was as anxious as I to see his handiwork.

My mummy wrapping was cut off and I saw a tight, slim, young-looking neck. My face was a disaster, but not as bad as expected. The tightness of my throat area hadn't been the bandage, as I'd thought. It was my own tight muscles and skin. Unbelievable!

My head was rebandaged like a nun's of yesteryear, no hair showing. I tied on a scarf,

put on my robe and dark glasses, and left the hospital on my husband's arm.

I'd been warned not to talk, lift my chin, turn my head, chew, laugh, or cry, but all I wanted to do was sleep that first week.

Later, I learned I'd received only sufficient general anaesthetic to totally deaden the surgical area. Then I was held in a non-remembering state for the duration of the operation. Whatever they used caused lethargy for fifteen days. Loss of blood caused a weakness that persisted beyond the fourth week.

My projects lay untouched while I rested, husbanding my energies for as small an effort as holding a book. I turned my head with my hands to protect my weak neck muscles, and moved very slowly when moving was necessary.

Five days after surgery I visited Dr. B for a check-up and change of bandage. The size of the blood clots in my ears amazed my husband. No wonder I'd seemed deaf.

All of my bandages and some of my stitches were removed after seven days, and my doctor prescribed a white scarf for a headcovering. Colored dyes could prove harmful.

At last I could shampoo my hair, a major undertaking since dried blood caked my short, fine hair. Shampooing twice in the shower barely began the task, so I surrendered. My husband finished the cleaning/combing routine with me draped over the kitchen sink. Seeing hair again was pleasant, but wiry stitches stuck out from the sides of my head and both ears and scalp were tender. I was pleased to note the doctor hadn't plowed a wide, naked trail but had made neat, nearly-invisible stitches. I'd not realized that a Face Lift enlarges facial area and decreases hair area. My losing *any* hair is a catastrophe.

Since I'd had facial surgery at my life-time's lowest weight I could look down at slim legs and gain some comfort. I needed lots of comfort, for my face looked like a monkey's. Makeup would have helped, but since my face was still tender that camouflage was denied me. It was difficult to sit still, look awful, and be forbidden to improve my appearance.

During the long second week I began to identify some of my downs. The image in the mirror which typically smiled back at me was gone. In her place I saw a zombie. Her face was frozen and her eyes, the same green as mine, stared back from a distorted face that bore no other resemblance.

Losing one's visual identity hurts. My face was thick ear-to-ear. My hair fell out . . . doubtless from the anesthesia . . . I should have expected this since it happened after both children were born. As soon as my strength returned, I headed for the nearest wig counter.

My downs took place even though I knew I was progressing nicely, even though my family comforted me.

My surgeon gave me a nice "up" feeling on the eleventh day. He found I was healing ahead of schedule on the right side, less swelling there, and healing normally on the left. The rest of the stitches came out and we all congratulated ourselves that I wasn't too bruised. Stitch removal seemed similar in pain to an ineptly wielded hypodermic needle.

Doctor B showed my husband and me a diagram of facial muscles and explained what the muscle tightening part of the surgery entailed. We'd been curious. After making the incisions, the doctor attached the sides of the broad thin sheet of muscle which extends downward from the jaw and chin to the facia or lining of the mastoid. He, in effect, tightened the sling of muscles which gives one a youthful neck.

Next he picked up two muscle groups, one beside the mouth, the other at the hollow of the cheek. He shortened these and reattached them to the areas in front of my ears.

Excess neck skin (by now almost one and one-fourth inches) was lifted up and into a two-inch horizontal incision in my hair behind each ear. Facial skin was lifted and tightened as high as my forehead, and extra skin (nearly one inch of it) was excised via vertical incisions in the hair above my ears.

To smooth my face Doctor B made careful incisions in front of each ear. Going inside my ears for the center part, he continued below the lobe and upwards to the horizontal incision. Now he removed loose skin. My scars weren't noticeable from the very beginning unless I looked for them. Only my hair dresser knows for sure that I've had a Lift.

The third week inched by. Doctor B checked my scars, photographed me, then showed me my unbecoming "before" pictures. Joy! That was me no longer. I could use makeup, hats, wigs, exercise carefully, and do anything I felt up to. I made an appointment to return in six weeks and hoped to look my "new" "normal" self by then.

My first time in public was physically wearing, and the same comment came from everyone who spoke, "You look as though you've lost weight!" No one looked at me strangely.

At four weeks I still walked slowly to conserve my limited energy, but I was no longer hybernating. My schedule included light shopping and luncheon with a friend, an evening meeting (for which I rested most of the day), an early dinner and movie, plus, incidentally, doing two television appearances.

The effect of my "new" look on my husband astonished me. He'd married a plain girl, but now she wasn't plain. This sufficiently disturbed him to force a rethinking of our relationship. His conclusion was one I'd always known. He was man enough to hold a pretty wife.

One year after surgery I felt as though the Face Lift had happened to someone else. Surely I'd always had smooth, tight skin. A perceptive friend commented, "At last your face matches your interior. That unattractive mask you wore has been removed."

Although this Face Lift concerned a woman, men have increasingly adopted such procedures as well as many of the ones which follow in the next chapter,

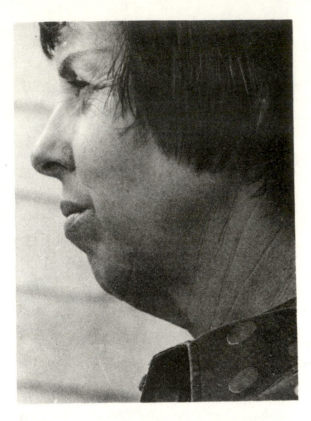

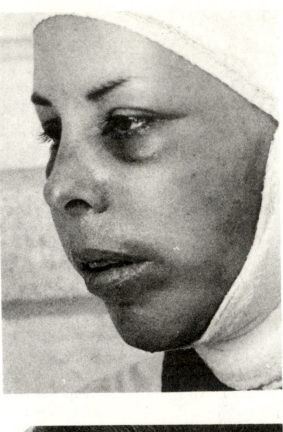

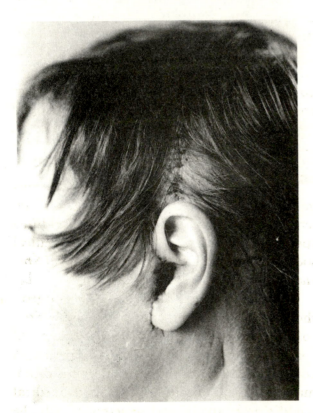

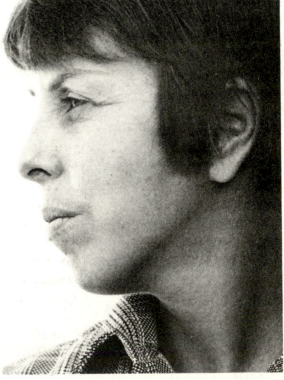

1. Before surgery
   2. The worst (one day after)
3. The scar
   4. Three weeks after

## 26

Your Visible Problems

When a detail of your appearance blocks you, makes you feel devalued, don't give up. Do something. Find out if corrective surgery is desirable medically, financially and psychologically. If surgery is the answer, do it. If it isn't, accept that feature as an interesting uniqueness and turn your attention toward living.

Reconstructive and cosmetic surgeons are careful to screen prospective patients, eliminating those with unrealistic expectations. Plastic surgery won't make you a corporate bigwig if you haven't the talent, training and perseverance. It won't make you the life of the party if you haven't the energy and personality. It won't make the one-you-love love you more. At best, cosmetic surgery can modify your looks, but it can't solve all your problems.

If you are contemplating this type of surgery, ask yourself the following questions:

Would an inner change do me more good than an outer one? _____ yes _____ no

What do I expect this change will do for me and my life? _____

Can I honestly expect changing my_____ will alter my life in the way I hope? _____yes _____no

Am I looking for an easy way out of a difficult situation? _____yes _____ no

Is improving my appearance worth the inconvenience, possible pain and cost? _____yes _____no

Can I handle the psychological adjustment? _____yes _____no

Be warned—even if you pass this test to your satisfaction—surgery carries with it discomfort if not actual pain. Those with low pain thresholds should consider carefully. One's pocketbook can be pained, as well; for unless surgery's classified "corrective" to repair past damage or improve your health, medical insurance doesn't cover it.

Surgeons don't guarantee you'll receive the nose-you-pine-for, either. They work with existing bone structure and features to construct what *they* feel becomes you.

Ultimately, cosmetic surgery is a tradeoff. You keep your old features and skin with *no* scars or gain better features, smoother areas or tighter skin with pain and scarring.

— SQUARE ONE —

Consult with a *qualified* cosmetic surgeon. There are several ways to locate one: referral by your physician, listing of qualified specialists from your hospital or medical society, or listing in *Directory of Medical Specialists* in your public library.

The person you choose as your surgeon should be a trusted parent, friend, and white-coated medical specialist between forty and sixty years old—of an age to be experienced yet aware of new techniques. Check his diplomas. They'll indicate his age plus medical schools and professional societies. Ideally, he should be a member of the American Society of Plastic and Reconstructive Surgeons or the American Association of Cosmetic Surgeons.

During your initial consultation, the surgeon will take a medical history, ask what you're interested in changing, and give you a brief examination. He may show before-and-after slides of patients who've had your contemplated surgery, although many surgeons do not. He'll get some feel for your reasons for requesting change and give specific information about hospitalization, anaesthetic, incisions, recovery time, amount of pain, potential hazards and costs.

Don't be disappointed if he decides surgery isn't your solution. He's saving you money, time, pain and future disappointment. On the other hand, check with another specialist if you feel the first doctor's response is biased, his approach raises questions, his fee's too high, or if you aren't simpatico.

Since cosmetic and reconstruction surgery covers a wide range of problems, only a brief description of the most common will be attempted.

— WINNING BY A NOSE —

Pat qualified many of her statements with disparaging comments about her nose. "Yes, the glasses look okay, but no glasses look great with this nose centering them." Another time, "No hairdo works with my nose!" Hers wasn't a Cyrano nose either, just one slightly wider and heavier than seemed appropriate for her slender face. She seemed constantly aware of it—the rest of us unaware. We'd accepted Pat's features and never thought of them—thought, instead, of her kindness.

Pat was in her late thirties before she had her Nose Reconstructed, but noses can be done as soon as bone structure is mature, as early as one's fifteenth birthday. Thin, hooked noses are relatively easy to correct. Thick, bulbous noses with heavy, large-pored skin are more difficult. Button or hollow noses may require silicone implants.

Pat's nose was reshaped through the nostrils to eliminate scars, but narrowing the nostril area necessitated exterior incisions and tiny stitches along the nostril folds.

Nose surgery is generally one to two hours. Hospitalization is two to three nights. Surgeons prefer using a local anesthesia, but "generals" are sometimes given. Reconstructed noses may be packed, splinted, and bandaged for as long as twelve days, after which time the nose begins to take on its new appearance. Swelling and eye area discoloration disappear after two or three weeks, but it takes six to ten months before the nose reaches its final shape.

This type of surgery costs between $500 and $2,000 plus anesthesia and hospitalization. Pat could claim most of the expense on her medical insurance as the surgeon found her nose had been broken in childhood.

Before you commit your nose to a surgeon, see samples of his work or meet his former patients. The nose he's put on fifty other patients can't be right for you. Each nose should be tailored to the face and body it graces, not to the doctor's or your ideal in noses.

Pat told me some time after surgery, "My new, elegant nose is somewhat less efficient than the old one, for the air passages were narrowed—but I love it!"

— KEEPING YOUR CHIN UP —

Lynn, handsome as a model, surprised us with the fact that he'd once had no chin, just a mouth-to-neck slope. Unbelievable. There were no scars, no evidence of surgery, yet his jawline looked great. How did they do it?

A competent surgeon formed a pocket in Lynn's chin via a small incision inside his mouth between lower lip and gums. Into this pocket he slipped a silicone wedge. This wedge was carefully selected to enhance Lynn's facial bone structure. The opening was sutured. Two hazards remained: infection and dislocation. To forestall infection, Lynn's surgeon prescribed gargling with warm saltwater. To insure that the wedge didn't slip from its preferred seat Lynn was asked to keep his jaw in a fixed position for nearly two weeks while scar tissue built-up around the silicone. Limited talking and a liquid diet—ugh!

150

Lynn's surgery was performed in a hospital, as an outpatient. His anaesthesia was local—the operation over in less than an hour. Swelling and discoloration were worse than he anticipated, but they faded in a little over two weeks. He was completely recovered in six months.

When asked if it hurt, Lynn said, "About as much as having a couple of impacted wisdom teeth extracted." It was obviously worth it. His profile is Grecian.

Marilyn Monroe was unsuccessful in Hollywood because of an inadequate chin projection. This was before the age of silicone implants, but her chin was augmented anyway—with hipbone. The rest is history.

Every chin problem may not be solved as easily as Lynn's nor with the difficulty of Marilyn's. Chin Reduction requires bone removal, sometimes breaking the jawbone and resetting the jaw in better alignment using steel sutures.

When upper and lower teeth don't align, either upper or lower jaw can be broken and shifted—big help to the profile as well as one's chewing capacity. Check with your orthopedic surgeon about this.

Chin reshaping can cost from $350 to $2,500, depending upon the complexity of the problem and the renown of the surgeon.

— EYE, THAT'S THE PROBLEM —

Bags under the eyes a problem of the aging? Yes, but not always. Chris was barely sixteen, but her undereye luggage was impressive. Cause? Heredity. She'd inherited a weak septum orbitale which permitted herniation of the underlying fat. Solution? Surgery.

A neat incision was made directly below Chris's lower lashes. Excess fat was removed and the opening was closed with stitches. Like Lynn's chin, Chris's "bags" were removed under local anaesthetic and relatively quickly. Many doctors require no postoperative bandages, just a pair of dark glasses for protection, but Lynn's surgeon used a tape to control swelling and possible bleeding. Stitches were removed in six days, and two weeks later she looked better than new.

A number of systemic problems, including edema, cause puffiness, so all "bags" may not require surgery. Have a careful physical *before* you see a surgeon.

Another common eye problem occurs when a hood of excess eyelid skin lays in folds on the upper lashes, blocking upward vision, weighting down the eye, and aging the appearance. Unlike lower eye surgery, upper eye surgery can be claimed on most medical insurance policies as correction of a visual handicap.

Upper incisions are made in the natural creases of the lid, excess skin and any superfluous fat is removed and the whole sutured. Upper surgery alone may cost as little as $500. Adding lower eye surgery would make your bill higher. Both together will cost between $1,000 and $1,500 plus hospitalization. Hospitalization is usually just the cost of the operating room plus drugs and supplies—not overnight.

— CAREFUL, KISSING ZONE —

Robert felt ashamed. Being a teenager was hard enough, but to have *thick lips* was terrible. No girl would look at him. He wanted to chuck school, home, everything. Instead, he saw a cosmetic surgeon and found a new smile.

The surgeon cut a section from the inside of each lip, rolling the lip inward. Care had to be taken not to excise too much or Robert's mouth wouldn't close. His lips swelled and hurt and he couldn't see the results for over two weeks, but slowly new lips emerged. They were worth everything.

Normal cost for Lip Reduction is $250 to $600 plus hospitalization. Surgery to correct drooping lips or other flaws that require external stitches are usually discouraged— scars would be worse than the problem.

— WINDFLAPS —

Bing Crosby was a success despite Dumbo ears and so was Clark Gable. It can be done, but it isn't necessary. Protruding ears can be corrected any time after one's seventh birthday. Reduction of Ear Size and/or Reduction of Earlobe Size may require two nights' hospitalization or can be done on an outpatient basis. Children are given general anaesthetics, but a local is sufficient for adults. Bandages are removed in approximately seven days, stitches are out in two weeks and the patient sleeps with a scarf covering the ears for several months. Cost is $500 to $1,250 plus hospitalization.

Blacks who have been disfigured by keloidal scar buildup following earpiercing can also find surgical help. New techniques excise the keloid and reshape the earlobe. Post operative procedures of cortisone injections and/or X-ray treatments prevent recurrence.

— BUSTY OR BUSTED —

Breasts can be firmed, reshaped, replaced, enlarged, or reduced by cosmetic surgery. For simplicity, we'll deal only with enlargement and reduction.

Most common candidates for Breast Reduction Surgery are forty-plus year old women with large breasts. They have endured postural problems, back pain, fungus infections under the breasts, painfully grooved shoulders from bra strap pull, or even constricted breathing caused by excess weight on the chest. But their younger sisters, suffering embarrassment and difficulty in finding clothing, also seek relief. An added incentive to both may be the higher breast cancer risk for women with large breasts.

Reduction surgery takes place in three steps. First, the nipple and aureola are repositioned higher on the breast. Second, the excessive mass of skin and tissue is removed. Third, the surrounding skin is reshaped.

Scarring is inevitable, but many women are willing to exchange a large unscarred breast for a small, shapely scarred one. And with the passage of time such scars usually become flat and less noticeable.

Retaining the ability to breastfeed an infant depends upon the manner in which the nipple was moved, the amount of necessary reduction and how young the patient. Despite its handicaps, women who have undergone Breast Reduction Surgery are among the most satisfied patients of all those having cosmetic surgery.

With Reduction Surgery, count on five to seven days in the hospital, a general anaesthetic, and an operation lasting two and one-half to five hours. There is more discomfort than for those having augmentation surgery beause more tissue is involved. You leave the hospital heavily bandaged and your activities are limited for four to six weeks. Fees, determined by the complexity of your problem and your ability to pay, vary from $1,000 to $3,000 plus hospitalization.

Unlike Breast Reductions, most Breast Enlargement Surgery is done in the late teens or twenties. An incision is made under the breast, and a silicone implant is positioned behind the natural breast tissue to lift and firm it. This Augmentation Surgery takes about an hour and can be performed on an outpatient basis with local anaesthesia and sedation if the patient isn't overly nervous, otherwise it requires hospitalization and a general anaesthetic.

Your doctor will choose from several different materials and shapes. Trust him. But NEVER let anyone "inject" you with silicone! Silicone injection can cause death, disintegration of the breasts, fullness displaced to another, less desirable location in the body, or problems necessitating breast amputation. Scary!

Augmentation Surgery fees average between $1,000 and $2,000 plus cost of the implants, hospitalization and anaesthesiologist. Implants cost $200 to $300.

Most patients experience some muscle spasm and pain during the twenty-four hours following surgery, but medication relieves them. For the first two to three weeks you refrain from jerky or heavy lifting type activities. During the second two week period, you may drive, type and perform other moderate chores. At the end of the month all normal activity may be resumed, including strenuous sports.

— NEED A-PEEL? —

Although life begins at forty in other respects, your face seems to give-up about that age and lines, wrinkles, and sag begin to take over. Eyelid surgery as well as face and neck lifting can help the aging face, but additional help is often needed and surgeons differ in recommendations as well as order of procedure.

Basically, two techniques are used to improve facial tone and texture: Chemical Peel (including Dermabrasion) and Face Lifts (previously discussed).

Dermabrasion works best for acne and laceration scars. It, like a Chemical Peel, removes your outer skin layers but is controlled mechanically (as a file removes), not chemically (as an acid removes).

Chemical Peel is suggested for those, like Betty, who have considerable wrinkling and/or frown lines, yet whose skin is fairly tight. The Peel is often suggested following a Face Lift, to remove surface scars, to correct weathered, leathery skin and for deep lines around the mouth. Men, because of their beards, aren't candidates for this procedure.

Betty entered the hospital one night before her Peel and was tranquilized immediately before the procedure. Exposed portions of her face, into the hairline and onto her lips, were treated with a chemical. Then her face was covered with a special waterproof adhesive tape that remained in place for thirty-six hours as an essential part of the process.

On removal of the tape, Betty's face was powdered with a face-drying chemical which produced an overall scab. The scab gradually separated over a period of days, and her exposed skin flamed scarlet and felt pebbly. A further treatment, this time a cream, reduced the red to a milk pink tone which remained for nearly six months. Opaque makeup hid the pinkness after the ninth day, but it took more than two weeks before Betty could be comfortable with her new face at a party. One doesn't flaunt a severe burn.

Sunlight and birth control pills can cause unattractive discoloration of delicate new skin, so both were forbidden for six months following the Peel.

Fee for a Chemical Peel is $500 to $2,000 plus one to two nights of hospital expense. Neither Eyelid Surgery nor the Face Lift is as emotionally demanding and discomforting to a patient as the Chemical Peel. For a period of time you look horrible!

— IN GENERAL —

Cosmetic or Aesthetic Surgery is surface surgery and patients in otherwise good health can tolerate several hours in the operating room. This may allow more than one surgical procedure and save you work-time and hospital expense. Imagine coming out of the hospital with less here, more there! Ask your surgeon about combining procedures.

Ask your surgeon, too, about the more exotic surgical procedures which include Buttocks Augmentation, Buttocks and Thigh Reduction, Arm Reduction, Abdominoplasty (the tummy tuck), and implant procedures for male impotence. All are becoming increasingly common and producing fine results. Needless to say, if any of these problems can be corrected by psychological help, diet or exercise, do so. But if they can't, there are surgical answers.

Candidates for Cosmetic Surgery should be healthy and slim. Doctors are loath to work on anyone overweight or with poor skin due to smoking, drinking or improper diet. The finished product is only as good as the material you supply, so get your act together! Love yourself into good health. You know how.

Should YOU have Cosmetic Surgery? Only you can say. *How you react to what you see in the mirror is far more important than what is actually there.*

Why is information about the non-visible included in a book called LOOK LIKE YOURSELF & LOVE IT!? You'll find the answer in this last chapter.

27

Your Non-visible Self

You've mastered your "look" and aligned both weight and posture. Congratulations! The mirror undoubtedly corroborates what you smilingly know—YOU LOOK SMASH-ING! So why a chapter on the non-visible?

Others see you differently than does your mirror. They see your:

— MOVEMENT —

As you learned in chapter 16, good posture flatters your figure and whittles pounds off your appearance, but that's not all. Good posture also aids circulation, protects your back from strain and allows you to stand and move efficiently and gracefully. Reread the seven steps To Improve Your Posture on page 96. Then . . .

When You Walk, align your torso before stepping off with an easy stride, legs swinging from your hip sockets. Feel as though you're leading with your thighs—walk with hands on thighs until you get the feel. Push off with the big toe of your rear foot, shift your weight to the heel-ball-toe of the forward foot, repeat. Walk lightly, with feet close together, pointed ahead, and just skimming the floor.

Check your shoulders. You want them perfectly still with relaxed arms and fingertips just brushing your sides. Motionless buttocks are the goal.

When You Stand, relax your knees. Women look most graceful in the "model's stance," leading foot pointing straight ahead, the rear foot at an angle with its ball one and

one-half inches from the heel of the front foot. Now it's easy to transfer weight from foot to foot.

To avoid a dejected simian illusion, keep at least one hand at waist level, or above, at all times. Be sure no body line droops.

When You Sit, choose a straight chair with a firm seat. Approach; turn; feel the front edge of the seat with the back of one leg. Keeping buttocks tucked under, lower yourself to the seat edge, then ease back.

Never cross your legs when on a platform, on display, or if you have large legs or thighs. Graceful women slant their legs to one side with feet crossed and form elongated lines with their hands.

To arise from a chair, push forward to the seat edge by pressing against the chairback with your shoulders. With one foot ahead of the other and an upright torso, gently rise.

Upon entering a car, turn your back to the seat, lower yourself to the seat edge, ease back, and (keeping feet together) swing both legs inside. It's much like sitting in a chair.

Leaving a car is just the reverse. Feet come out together. You slide your body to the seat edge and arise. *While in the car sit with your whole back touching the seat.*

When You Climb Stairs, let thigh and leg muscles do the work. Keep your knees bent and torso erect. There should be no bouncing. One hand at waist level adds grace. If you must look at the stairs while descending, glance over your shoulders. Dropping the

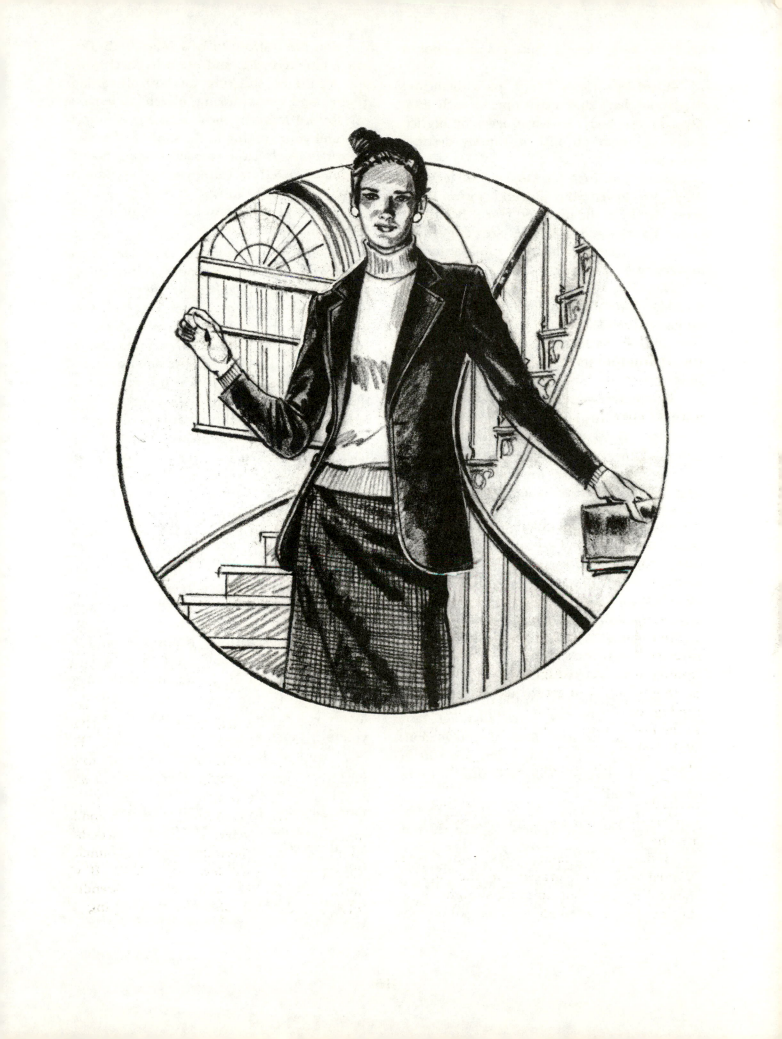

head to look throws buttocks out—not a pretty sight.

When You Carry Loads, pack them into two equal bags and carry one in each arm, close to the body, at waist level or higher. Propping them on hip or tummy destroys symmetry.

When You Pick-Up Objects, use legs and thighs to lower your upright torso. Don't bend over from the hips and reach. Bend your knees. Your large leg muscles are designed for lifting . . . your back isn't . . . and the former movement is graceful.

Handling a Coat To put on—relax your shoulders.Slip one arm deep into a sleeve; the opposite shoulder must remain level with arm only slightly backward. Smoothly slide your second arm into its sleeve. Adjust the shoulder area.

To remove—grasp lapels and slip the front slightly upwards and back to free your shoulders. Drop one arm and let your coat fall, pivoting it on the arm still encased. With your free hand, grasp the coat's neckline at your still-covered arm and lift, slipping the second arm free.

Now, with suggestions for graceful movements in mind—practice. Practice when you're alone and when you're with others. Practice until graceful movement becomes your nature. Pretending that *you're watched every moment* can change the way you move. See if it helps. You *can* move gracefully—do it!

— SPEECH —

Those meeting you for the first time automatically note your sex, personality, age, taste and apparent income. And, if you've done your homework, the image they see will be honest and attractive. You look fine, but how do you sound?

Pretty, Type-One, Mary Beth looked luscious. Her face and frame delighted the eye, but eligible males—hurrying to her side— braked when she spoke. Shrill voice and constant giggle outraged the ear. Mary Beth was unaware of her vocal problems. She'd never heard herself.

You can't afford to be a Mary Beth. Borrow a tape recorder, and use it to check yourself. You'll be checking for both discordant quality and embarrassing speech patterns.

Record a family meal, a phone conversation and your singing in the shower or behind the car's wheel. Tape yourself reading poetry, talking to a fellow employee and communicating with your boss.

Find a private place for listening to your collection. Take notes.

Is your voice resonant? Confident? Pleasant? Are your speech patterns interesting? Your vocabulary rich? Your interplay with others sensitive? Is your pitch pleasant, your volume appropriate to the circumstances? Are your words clear, your conversation free of "ughs," "you knows," giggles and apologies? Do your words and sentences inflect *down*, as though you mean what you say, or *up*, registering uncertainty and tentativeness? Do you accept or reject compliments? Can you spot lack of confidence in, "It's nice, *don't you think?*" "*Isn't that right, dear?*" and "*Just ask my friend, he'll tell you.*"? Is your outlook sunny or whiney and doomsday?

The vocal problems you've noted can be solved and you'll want to solve them quickly once you hear yourself. Causing a listener discomfort is no one's preference.

If you suspect your pitch is too high, repeat a short sentence such as, "Come on," "Let's go," several times. If possible, hold the tone of the last syllable while you find the identical pitch on the piano. Women's voices sound best in the vicinity of "middle C." Men's voices sound best an octave lower. If you're as much as four notes higher than your "C," work at lowering your pitch. Dorothy Sarnoff's classic paperback, *Speech Can Change Your Life*, will help you attain a more pleasing pitch if you'll read it.

Improving your speech isn't difficult. Good speech books, such as the one mentioned, can also help with other vocal problems. You can work with a qualified speech consultant/therapist or enroll in a speech course that uses video-tape. Seeing yourself as you talk grooms body language along with your voice.

What to say can pose problems, but the solution isn't difficult—merely read as widely as possible. A well-written newspaper can be your best ally if you read it daily.

Practice active listening. Care enough about your conversational partner to consider what he/she's feeling and saying. Encourage sharing by both of you. Any interchange which doesn't allow time for both to talk is dissatisfying.

Do your homework well ahead of speeches, lectures and workshops. Several good speech-preparation books are listed in the Appendix.

— TIME PLANNING SKILLS —

When reading the words, *time planning* do you automatically think of: (check one)
- a- A job for every minute.
- b- Guilt.
- c- I'm a pendulum swinging between *a* and *b*.
- d- It helps me to accomplish important goals without pressure.

If you checked *a, b* or *c*, consider reading time consultant Allen Lakein's excellent paperback, *How to Get Control of Your Time and Your Life*. He'll help you to set goals, creatively structure your time, and erase the discrepancy between the things you do and those you want to do. Both the pressured executive and a person with few responsibilities can benefit.

Incorporating data from *this* book into your lifestyle requires reorganization, and time planning is the easiest way to gain the extra time and order you need for constructive change.

Remember, *bad habits can be exchanged for good ones*. Everytime you go against a habit you weaken that habit. But you also weaken the power of your other bad habits as well—making them easier to break. Everytime you use your will to control what you do, you develop additional control. And when strong, this control can be channeled in any direction you decide.

— JOB SATISFACTION —

Do you like your occupation? Some individuals love their work; other punish themselves, daily, with jobs they detest. Not surprisingly, the former work easily and efficiently; the latter expend great energy yet accomplish little.

Studies, begun in 1922, by the Johnson O'Connor Research Foundation have long proved the existence of "innate abilities." These are inherited aptitudes (natural talents or abilities) which you can't change, no matter the effort expended. You either have a knack with an artist's pencil or you don't.

Individuals have differing abilities, and two people who share the same aptitude will display varying degrees of skill in it. Through testing, abilities can be measured, but what's the purpose?

By understanding your strengths and weaknesses you gain insight into previous successes and failures. You stop expecting more of yourself in certain areas than you're capable of delivering. And by matching your profile of highs and lows to those of successful individuals you can discover the vocation in which you have the aptitudes for success.

All doctors who are happy in their work will have nearly-identical patterns of highs and lows on aptitude tests. So will all salesmen, all teachers, all foresters, and all artists.

Don't worry that you have insufficient talents. The person with few abilities is the easiest person to place in the perfect job. The person with too-many aptitudes is the one with career problems. Entrepreneurship is one vocation with sufficient variety to interest the multi-talented person. It was the choice of your author.

An unused talent will cause you restlessness or unhappiness even though you're ideally situated in all other respects. Discover your abilities and use them all in either your work or your free time.

Is a large vocabulary important? It certainly is. And, unlike aptitudes, skill with words can be changed. Read widely, study word derivations and associate with those having extensive vocabularies. The top person in any field is the one with the best grasp of language. You can be that person.

If you hate your present job and see no alternative, contact the Johnson O'Connor Research Foundation nearest you. There are twelve in the United States, all listed in the Appendix. If your son or daughter hasn't decided on a career and needs to, have them tested. Knowing the profession in which they can succeed is fine insurance against vocational detours, and aptitudes are set by age fourteen.

A less expensive—but also less direct—means of finding your ideal profession can come through reading the bestselling paperback, *What Color Is Your Parachute?* A workbook entitled *Where Do I Go From Here With My Life* and a course have been developed to supplement the basic information. They are also listed in the Appendix.

Seek a satisfying vocation. Pay the price of necessary change. Life is too short to spend it doing something you hate. Your satisfaction or dissastisfaction will build or destroy relationships and leave happy or disgruntled lines on your face.

— INTERIOR GROWTH —

Have you ever known a paragon—someone who did, said, looked exactly right at all time? How did you feel about him/her? Were you cozy friends or distant and evaluative?

The "perfect" person, fearing exposure, sacrifices spontaneity and naturalness for a flawless image. Observers react competitively or with reserve, only loving the paragon when flaws are glimpsed. The answer is, of course . . . be loveable . . . be yourself.

Maturity brings a healthy sense of self, but it isn't a gift of years; maturity comes when you choose to grow-up and take steps to do so.

Some questions for evaluating your present stage of maturity include:

Are YOU responsible for your emotions and actions? Others can't make you angry or happy. YOU are the one who chooses anger or happiness.

Do you ACCEPT problems and change? These are catalysts which help you grow. Often frightening and sometimes painful, they shouldn't be fought. The happiest and best-adjusted individuals are those who accept change.

What are your motives? Are the actions you choose satisfying in the doing, or do you get your "gold stars" from the approval of others? Choose projects which don't require "strokes" from others to be enjoyable.

Why pamper yourself? It saves you from martyrdom. Spend time, daily, on activities you enjoy; they'll brighten each day as well as your life.

Is each moment lived fully? This minute is the only one you can live. Don't wait; live now. The past and future are unattainable—the present is priceless.

Are you transparent? Do you express (in terms of how you feel) your hurt, joy, disappointment, love to those you care about? It takes courage to expose yourself, but from such exposure come the richest relationships.

Do you consider those close to you as "loaned?" They aren't your possessions, nor do you have a guarantee you'll have them close to you next year. Enjoy each moment of their company, and love them while you can. The loss of a child, parent or spouse needn't produce anger or guilt. It needs acceptance as a part of living.

Can he/she be EVERYTHING to you? No. You and your loved one are like twin pomander balls—oranges stuck round with cloves. When you're together, a number of the cloves match-up. The longer you work together in the relationship the more common areas you connect. But, since the cloves on the backs of both oranges will never touch, don't expect them to. Each of you need others for completion in non-connected areas.

Have you a source of comfort, answers and identity? The longing, aching loneliness you feel and everyone feels can't be cured by another person. And expecting a love-partner to satisfy your hunger is both unfair and destructive.

Only One can love you wholly, forgive you totally, and fill you with a sustaining peace. Seek Him.

"God does not die on the day when we cease to believe in a personal diety, but we die on the day when our lives cease to be illumined by the steady radiance, renewed daily, of a wonder, the source of which is beyond reason."

Dag Hammarskjold - *Markings*
Translated from the Swedish by Leif Sjoberg & W. H. Auden, Alfred A. Knopf, Inc., 1964.

Appendix

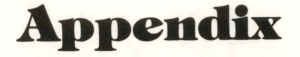

Various authors and services have been influential in developing my "look" and my feelings about myself. With hope that they may also help you, I list them.

— AUTHORS —

Tim LaHaye's *Spirit Controlled Temperament*, Tyndale, 1966. *Transformed Temperaments*, Tyndale, 1971. *Understanding The Male Temperament*, Revell, 1977.

Beverly LaHaye's *Spirit-Controlled Woman*, Harvest House, 1976, plus this couple's other writings.

John T. Molloy's *Dress For Success*, Warner Books, 1978. *Woman's Dress For Success*, Warner Books, 1978.

Glamour's *Success Book*, Conde Naste Publications, 1979.

Charles Hix's *Looking Good, A Guide For Men*, Pocket Books, 1978, and *Dressing Right*, St. Martin's Press, 1978.

Peter Carlsen and William Wilson's *Man-Style*, Clarkson N. Potter, Inc., 1977.

Nikki & David Goldbeck's *The Dieter's Companion*, McGraw-Hill, 1975.

Theodore Berland and Consumer Guide's *Rating The Diets*, Beekman House, 1979.

Deborah Szekely Mazzanti's *Secrets Of The Golden Door*, William Morrow, 1977, wonderful recipes!

Charles T. Kuntzlemann & Editors of Consumers Guide's *Rating The Exercises*, 1978.

Marjorie Craig's *Miss Craig's 21-Day Shape-Up Program For Men And Women*, Random House, 1968.

Kenneth H. Cooper, M.D.'s *Aerobics*, M. Evans & Co., 1968. *The Aerobic Way*, Bantam, 1978.

Mildred Cooper & Kenneth Cooper's *Aerobics For Women*, Bantam, 1973.

Dr. Carl Kenyon's *How To Avoid Rip-offs At The Dentist*, Sovereign Books, 1979.

Thomas H. Sternberg's *More Than Skin Deep*, Doubleday, 1970.

Joan Rattner Heilman, as editor of *Kenneth's Complete Book On Hair*, Dell, 1972.

Dorothy Sarnoff's *Speech Can Change Your Life*, Dell, 1972.

Sandy Linver's *Speak Easy*, Summit Books, 1978.

John Ott's *How To Write And Deliver a Speech*, Cornerstone, 1976.

Allen Lakein's *How To Get Control Of Your Time And Your Life*, McKay, 1973. New American Library, 1974.

Richard N. Bolle's *What Color Is Your Parachute?* Ten-Speed Press, 1978.

John C. Crystal and Richard Bolles' *Where Do I Go From Here With My Life?*, The Seabury Press, 1974.

Jess Lair, Ph.D.'s *"I Ain't Much Baby— But I'm All I Got"* Fawcett Paperback, 1978.

Hannah Whiteall Smith's *The Christian's Secret Of A Happy Life*, Revell, 1870, a Spire paperback.

Catherine Marshall's *Beyond Our Selves*, Avon, 1974, plus everything she's written.

C. S. Lewis's *The Screwtape Letters*, Macmillan, 1967, plus all his writings, including the *Chronicles Of Narnia*, a 7-book fantasy series for children of all ages, Macmillan, 1970.

Merlin Carother's *Power In Praise*, Logos, 1972, plus his other writings.

Oswald Chamber's *My Utmost For His Highest*, Dodd Mead, 1935, a daily devotional still being sold.

— SERVICES —

Personal assistance with colors, hair, makeup and clothing can be obtained through:

JANE SEGERSTROM'S 4-T WORK-SHOPS—coming to major cities as early as 1982. For information, contact Triad Interests, Inc., Dept. L, P. O. Box 42006, Houston, Texas 77042.

PERSONAL STYLE COUNSELORS, 1067 Norwood Avenue, Oakland, California 94610.

Help for problem skin may be found through:

JENEAL INTERNATIONAL—SKIN CORRECTION CENTERS, 2721 Hillcroft, Houston, Texas 77027.

Personal testing of innate abilities is available through the non-profit:

JOHNSON O'CONNOR RESEARCH FOUNDATION (alternate name, *HUMAN ENGINEERING LABORATORIES*) at the following addresses:

Atlanta - 3445 Peachtree Road, N.E., Suite 340, Atlanta, Georgia 30326.

Boston - 347 Beacon Street, Boston, Massachusetts 02116.

Chicago - 161 East Erie Street, Chicago, Illinois 60611.

Detroit - 27301 Dequindre, Suite 212, Madison Heights, Michigan 48071.

Fort Worth - 650 South Henderson Street, Fort Worth, Texas 76104.

Houston - 2055 South Gessner, Suite 124, Houston, Texas 77063.

Los Angeles - 611 South Catalina Street, Los Angeles, California 90005.

New York - 11 East 62nd Street, New York, New York 10021.

Philadelphia - 1518 Walnut Street, Suite 1409, Philadelphia, Pennsylvania 19102.

San Diego - 3004 Sixth Avenue, San Diego, California 92103.

Tulsa - 906 South Cheyenne Street, Tulsa, Oklahoma 74119.

Washington D.C. - 121 Second Street, N.E., Washington, D.C. 20002.

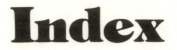

Index

166

Afterword

This book is designed as a tool to encourage and ease your transition from ordinary to WOW. I truly hope it succeeds.

But don't think its author is relaxing at some long-sought goal. I'm still learning, still refining my image—very aware that I'll never reach perfection, but the trip toward it has been wonderful, and there are exciting twists ahead.

My journey has led me from ill-health, excess weight, sedentary lifestyle, poor self-image, and lack of fashion sophistication to being younger, happier, more active, creative and beautiful than at any age of my life. I'm fifty years old, and it seems impossible.

Write to me if you have questions. I'll answer by mail, newsletter or column. Let me know, too, where I missed your needs or whatever you know that I should learn.

The very best wishes to you on your journey from what-you've-thought-you-were to what-you-can-become.

Jane Segerstrom

Jane Segerstrom
c/o Triad Press,
Dept. L
Post Office Box 42006
Houston, Texas 77042